NUTRITIONAL CARE for HIV-POSITIVE PERSONS:
A Manual for Individuals and Their Caregivers

NUTRITIONAL CARE for HIV-POSITIVE PERSONS:
A Manual for Individuals and Their Caregivers

Saroj M. Bahl, Ph.D., R.D., L.D.
Associate Professor
Department of Nutrition and Dietetics
School of Allied Health
The University of Texas-Houston
Health Science Center

and

James F. Hickson, Jr., Ph.D., R.D.
Retired
Adjunct Associate Professor
Division of Interdisciplinary Studies
School of Allied Health
The University of Texas-Houston
Health Science Center

CRC Press
Boca Raton   Ann Arbor   London   Tokyo

Library of Congress Cataloging-in-Publication Data

Bahl, Saroj M.
  Nutritional care for HIV-positive persons: a manual for individuals and their caregivers /
authors, Saroj M. Bahl and James Forbes Hickson, Jr.
      p.   cm. — (Modern nutrition)
  Includes bibliographical references and index.
  ISBN 0-8493-7843-5
  1. AIDS (Disease) — Diet therapy — Handbooks, manuals, etc. I. Hickson James F.,
1954-   . II. Title.   III. Series: Modern nutrition (Boca Raton, Florida)
RC607.A26B347   1994
616.97'920654—dc20   94-17805
                                                                                     CIP

© 1995 by CRC Press, Inc.

No claim to original U.S. Government works
International Standard Book Number 0-8493-7843-5
Library of Congress Card Number 94-17805
Printed in the United States of America 1 2 3 4 5 6 7 8 9 0
Printed on acid-free paper

SERIES PREFACE

The CRC Series in Modern Nutrition is dedicated to providing the widest possible coverage to topics in nutrition. Nutrition is an interdisciplinary, interprofessional field par excellance and is noted by its broad range and diversity. We trust that the titles and authorships in this series will reflect that range and diversity.

Published for a scholarly audience, the volumes of the Modern Nutrition series are designed to explain, review, and explore present knowledge and recent trends, developments, and advances in the field of nutrition. As such, they will also appeal to the educated layman. The format of the series will vary with the needs of individual authors and the topics, including, but not limited to, edited volumes, monographs, handbooks, and texts. Contributors from any bona fide area of nutrition, including the controversial, are welcome.

The contribution by S. Bahl and J.F. Hickson, *Nutritional Care for HIV-Positive Persons: A Manual for Individuals and Their Caregivers*, is a welcome addition to the series. The editors trust it will empower HIV-positive persons and their caregivers to utilize the best program of nutritional co-therapy possible.

A portion of the royalties from this volume will be donated to Omega House in Houston, an AIDS special care facility.

Ira Wolinsky, Ph.D.
James F. Hickson, Jr., Ph.D., R.D.
Series Editors

PREFACE

This book is a concise treatment of the principles, rules, and directions needed to address issues relating to diet and nutrition for persons living with the human immunodeficiency virus (HIV), the AIDS virus. We desire to empower you with practical, useful information that can be used to maximize your body's capacity to fight HIV infection and AIDS as well as to improve your quality of life when living with AIDS. To accomplish these objectives, we have mixed general discussion of selected topics with the "how to" specifics needed to take action on them.

This manual is aimed at two groups of persons: (1) those who are infected with HIV, with or without a diagnosis of AIDS, and (2) their caregivers, particularly those who have not been formally trained for the task. It is not directed to persons with a particular sexual preference or to the members of any one race, sex, or age group. Instead, we have been inclusive to reflect the spread of the disease into many segments of the American population including women, infants, and children.

As the numbers of infected persons has swelled, the time has come for an emphasis on practical rather than theoretical information. Many scholarly scientific and medical books and research articles have been published that describe AIDS as a disease process, what causes it, how it develops, its symptoms, and so on. We recognize the importance of defining AIDS and that it will be important to continue doing so in the future as new developments arise; however, the large and growing number of affected persons has created a burgeoning demand for a different kind of reading material.

Now there is a need for information with immediate usefulness, with direct application to people's daily lives. It is time for a manual that presents the facts, as we know them, with a minimum of interpretation or speculation. In addition, it is time for specific instructions regarding appropriate actions when they are known. Our perspective, to empower the reader with the information needed to take action, is very important because persons living with HIV and their caregivers should not have to interpret the meaning of scholarly books or research articles in order to learn how to proceed in the war against AIDS. We have tried, therefore, to design this manual to be used without guesswork.

Discussion and specifics for action regarding diet and nutrition have been firmly grounded in medical practice and scientific peer-reviewed literature in order to make it authoritative and reliable. However, we recognize that there are still many unknowns about HIV infection and AIDS. For this reason, we felt that it was important to balance traditional sources of information, observation, and practice with empirical or experiential perspectives (i.e., common experience). Accordingly, we have drawn heavily from our own professional experiences with persons with AIDS (PWAs) in City of Houston health care facilities and Texas Medical Center hospitals, as well as through personal interactions with health care professionals, including dietitians, physicians, and nurses, and caregivers and PWAs themselves.

While we have adopted a professional posture in our writing, the manual is not intended to follow a science or medical model. It was written for laymen, those persons who do not have specialized training in the jargon of science and medicine. Great care has been taken to pitch the language in terms that the reader will readily understand while still making an intelligent presentation. Hence, the wording reflects our high-wire attempt to strike a balance between simplicity and complexity. It was our objective that you would not need any specialized knowledge to read this book; the level we targeted was that of a home medical guide.

Our manual should not be confused with the many booklets and pamphlets that have already been written. Those publications are brief and simple treatments of minimal amounts of information. By contrast, the basic premise of this manual is to serve as a reference source by presenting a large, organized set of information in a concise fashion, without all the "bells and whistles".

We are very optimistic about the role that diet and nutrition can play for persons infected with HIV, especially those with AIDS who always seem to have diet-related difficulties of one kind or another. It seems ironic to us that there is much effort and resources being put into finding a cure, vaccines, and effective drug treatments, when the study of diet and nutrition at a fraction of the cost might hold considerable promise. Of course, diet and nutrition cannot be used to prevent or cure AIDS; however, there is a considerable body of experience regarding dietary behaviors and nutritional status to show that diet and nutrition can play a valuable role in the management of HIV infection and AIDS. We hope you will come to the same conclusion by reading and using this manual.

Saroj Bahl, Ph.D., R.D., L.D.
James F. Hickson, Jr., Ph.D., R.D.

THE AUTHORS

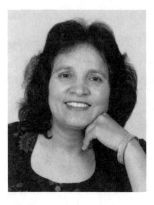

Saroj M. Bahl received her B.S. (Home Science), M.S. (Foods and Nutrition), and Ph.D. (Nutrition) degrees from Delhi University, India. She holds memberships in several professional societies, including the American Dietetic Association, Texas Dietetic Association, Society for Nutrition Education, Texas Society of Allied Health Professionals, and the American Institute of Life-Threatening Illness. Dr. Bahl has had extensive teaching experience, at both an undergraduate and graduate level. She has been the recipient of several awards for excellence in teaching, including the prestigious John P. McGovern Award of the University of Texas-Houston Health Science Center in 1992. Her other accomplishments include several scientific and educational publications in peer-reviewed journals, as well as over 50 presentations to professional and community groups. Dr. Bahl's specialty areas include nutrition education, curriculum development, and clinical nutrition with particular emphasis on maternal and child health. Nutritional concerns of pregnancy, lactation, infancy, and childhood constitute her major interests, and she has been involved with several hospitals and community clinics in the Harris County and Houston area in Texas.

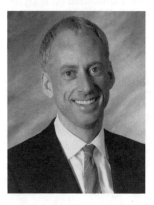

James F. Hickson, Jr., received his B.S. (Biochemistry) and Ph.D. (Human Nutrition, with a minor in Foods) degrees from Virginia Polytechnic Institute and State University in 1976 and 1980, respectively. He was formerly a faculty member at Indiana University, Bloomington, and the University of Texas Health Science Center at Houston. He is presently retired (1992) from the University of Texas system and is an adjunct associate professor at the University of Texas Health Science Center at Houston (1993). Dr. Hickson is a member of the American Dietetics Association, and he is also a registered dietitian through that organization. In addition, he is an emeritus member of the Institute of Food Technologists. Dr. Hickson was formerly a member of the American Institute for Nutrition, the American Society of Clinical Nutrition, and the honorary society Sigma Xi.

Dr. Hickson's specialties by his university training and experience are protein metabolism and exercise and amino acid analysis. At Indiana University, he and John E. Stockton designed one of the first programs for computerized dietary nutritional analysis (RECALL). This program was used to document and explain athletes' nutritional intakes. Throughout his 12 years as a university professor, Dr. Hickson's primary research efforts were directed toward the study of strength exercise (bodybuilding) on skeletal muscle tissue breakdown, the so-called "torn tissue" hypothesis.

In 1982, Dr. Hickson first took notice of what is now termed "AIDS". He sought to study nutritional connections and implications of this syndrome, before its etiology was linked directly to the human immunodeficiency virus (HIV). Sometime between 1988 and 1990, evidence began being reported by health care professionals that suggested a link between nutrition and morbidity (sickness) and mortality (death) in persons with AIDS. Learning this, Dr. Hickson began to make his own observations on PWAs and their nutritional habits and possible needs. He combined his knowledge with a thorough study of the research literature resulting in the chapters included in this text.

CONTENTS

Chapter 1

DIET AND NUTRITION FOR OPTIMAL IMMUNE FUNCTION

J. F. Hickson, Jr.

CONTENTS

I. INTRODUCTION

Poor diet and nutrition do not cause the acquired immunodeficiency syndrome (AIDS); it is caused by the human immunodeficiency virus (HIV). Yet, certain aspects of AIDS closely resemble the appearances of diseases resulting from essential nutrient deficiencies. Therefore, nutritional causes were proposed and investigated to explain AIDS when the first cases were reported in the early 1980s.

These early nutritional solutions to AIDS were reasonable in light of the body of scientific and medical knowledge at that time. First, there has been a historical link between malnutrition and infectious disease and death dating back for hundreds of years. Second, when cases of AIDS were first reported in the early 1980s, the direct involvement of certain nutrients in immune function was well established. Third, the nature of the virus causing AIDS had not been encountered previously, and scientists and physicians did not know to go looking for it. With the eventual discovery of HIV as the causative agent, nutrition lost favor as a factor to investigate.

Despite taking a back seat in regard to HIV as a causative agent in AIDS, poor diet and nutrition still remain the most important causes of impaired immune function around the world. In developing countries, immune status tends to be compromised by general starvation or the lack of food itself. In particular, the diet usually does not contain enough energy ("calories"), but a variety of vitamins and minerals as well as protein may also be missing.

It should be recognized that individuals in underdeveloped countries do not select a poor diet on purpose; they simply do not have the opportunity to achieve an adequate diet because food is not available, affordable, or present in sufficient variety. By contrast, in the industrialized countries, when nutrient deficiencies occur, they often are a result of unordinary dietary practices. Typically, deficiencies for individuals in the industrialized countries include one or a related group of micronutrients (i.e., minerals or vitamins). In summary, the peoples of industrialized and underdeveloped countries face different nutritional challenges.

Nutrients that play a particular role in immune function include vitamins A, B_2, B_6, biotin, folic acid, niacin, and pantothenic acid. All are required for maintenance of the integrity of the skin and lining of the gastrointestinal (GI) tract including the mouth, esophagus, stomach, and intestines. When these nutrients are deficient in the diet, then the integrity of the cells making up the skin barrier and GI tract lining (barrier) changes in such a way that microorganisms can pass across the barriers into the body.

With this exposure, an easy route of entry is made available to all types of microorganisms, including those that would not ordinarily cause disease in a healthy person. Once inside the body, these invaders cause illness in addition to that due to micronutrient deficiencies. This added layer of symptoms can mask the true, underlying cause of disease. Consequently, the infection is treated, but not the nutritional deficiency. Therefore, it is critical to be able to separate the effects of invading microbes from those of nutritional deficiencies in order to make the correct diagnosis and prescribe the correct treatment, as well as to understand and appreciate the role of nutrients in immune function.

II. ROLE OF SINGLE NUTRIENTS IN IMMUNITY

Today, deficiencies of single nutrients rarely occur in the modern, industrialized countries because food is plentiful, available, and affordable. Therefore, the information that has been gathered about deficiency syndromes is not based on the experience of the modern American population; instead, it has come from several other sources. Ironically, one of these was the study of Americans in the first half of the 20th century when nutritional disease was commonplace. More recently, malnourished peoples living in undeveloped countries around the world have been studied as the incidence of nutritional deficiency diseases disappeared in the United States and other industrialized countries.

A third approach yielding very specialized information has been the study of experimental animals fed custom diets lacking in specific nutrients. Animal studies provide important clues about the link between nutrition and immune function. However, they generally are of more academic interest than practical use because the results cannot be directly applied to people (animals are not people). The best approach would be to study humans in a controlled setting, but it would not be ethical to subject them to conditions that would surely compromise their health. Since human studies cannot be performed in most cases, animal studies fill a valuable gap. Nutrients implicated for roles in immune function include protein; vitamins A, E, B_2, B_6, and B_{12}; biotin; folic acid; niacin; pantothenic acid; iron; zinc; cadmium; calcium; chromium; copper; iodine; magnesium; manganese; and selenium. The need for energy also has been well established.

A. VITAMIN A

Vitamin A (retinol) was discovered in 1913 and given the curative property name "anti–infectious" vitamin. Although retinol has only recently been identified and synthesized in the laboratory, it has been known for many centuries as a component of certain foods. The role of retinol in immune function lies in the maintenance of the integrity of the skin and the lining of the GI tract as physical barriers to invasion by microorganisms. This is accomplished through control by the vitamin over the growth and development of the cells that make up the skin and GI lining.

It is exceptionally difficult to study the role of retinol in immune function because spontaneous (secondary) infections complicate the picture as soon as the deficiency state is achieved. It is difficult or impossible to know whether observations are the result of the vitamin deficiency or the infection. Therefore, what is known is largely based on studies of animals raised in germ–free (microbe–free) environments. It is of particular interest that the blood count of lymphocytes is reduced in retinol deficiency (Table 1). Loss of barrier integrity and decreased lymphocyte count are symptoms observed in AIDS.

TABLE 1
Changes in Immune Status with
Deficiencies of Selected Vitamins

Vitamin	Lymphocyte count	Antibody response	Skin, gut wall integrity
A (retinol)	PD	PD	C
B vitamins			
B$_2$ (riboflavin)	D	D	C
B$_6$ (pyridoxine)	PD	D	C
B$_{12}$ (cobalamine)	D	D	—
Biotin	—	PD	C
Folic acid	PD	PD	C
Niacin	—	—	C
Pantothenic acid	D	D	C
C (ascorbic acid)	PD	N	—
E (tocopherol)	D	D	—

Note: C = compromised, D = depression, PD = possible depression,
N = normal, dash (—) = no data or no effect.

B. B VITAMINS

Two factors of the immune system that often are mentioned in the context of AIDS are T lymphocytes and antibodies. The levels or responsiveness of these factors also undergo changes during deficiency of selected B vitamins, as shown in Table 1. However, since deficiencies of B vitamins do not all have the same effects, a range of responses is observed. For example, B$_1$ (thiamin) deficiency does not impair the immune system, while a lack of B$_6$ (pyridoxine) has a definite negative impact; biotin deficiency may or may not depress the antibody response.

Deficiencies of B vitamins are not likely to occur singly because these vitamins are found in many foods, usually together as a "complex". This makes it unusual for a deficiency to develop in the first place; even so, the fact that they appear together as a complex in foods makes it difficult to identify a deficiency unless telltale signs are observed in the patient, including anemia (folic acid, vitamin B$_{12}$), cream–colored, fatty stools (folic acid), unique skin pigmentation (niacin), nervous changes (vitamins B$_2$ and B$_{12}$), and others. What is most important to recognize is that deficiencies of several B vitamins induce disease symptoms resembling those of AIDS, especially the classic reduction in T lymphocyte count and the loss of GI tract integrity (Table 1).

1. Vitamin B$_2$

Vitamin B$_2$ (riboflavin) deficiency is associated with an increased suscep-tibility to microbial infection in several ways. There is a loss of GI tract integrity. In the healthy, normal individual, the skin and mucous membranes are physical barriers, preventing most microbes from getting through to the nutrient–rich blood on the other side. Furthermore, healthy tissues secrete factors with bactericidal action including fatty acids (skin), immunoglobulins (gut), acid (stomach), and enzymes (saliva). These defense mechanisms stop most microorganisms from invading the body.

In order for an invasion to proceed, there must be a "break" in the integrity of the system such as that which occurs with vitamin B_2 deficiency. The physical barrier is stripped away, leaving a raw surface and an exposed blood supply. Other factors also are lost, including the secretion of acid, enzymes, and immunoglobulins. The result is spontaneous infections that ordinarily would not occur in the healthy person with an intact immune system. In this way, B_2 deficiency resembles AIDS.

Riboflavin is also involved with the readiness of the immune system (i.e., the capacity to respond to a challenge). Ordinarily, modest levels of immune factors such as lymphocytes and antibodies are maintained circulating in the bloodstream. The levels of these factors are sufficient to mount a short–term challenge to invading microbes; however, many more immune factors are needed in a long–term challenge.

It takes energy to drive the enzymatic machinery that makes new immune factors, and vitamin B_2 is required to help produce that energy. In deficiency, the immune response is compromised in two ways by a lack of available energy. First, the capacity to respond to a long–term challenge is reduced because new immune factors cannot be synthesized in adequate amounts. Second, the circulating levels of immune factors, before any challenge, are below normal (Table 1). In other words, both responsiveness and readiness are compromised; therefore, B_2 deficiency resembles AIDS.

2. Vitamin B_6

Of all the B vitamins, B_6 (pyridoxine) has the most profound impact on immune status. The reason for its impact is that the processes of nucleic acid (deoxyribonucleic acid [DNA] and ribonucleic acid [RNA]) and protein syn-thesis, as well as cell multiplication, all require the vitamin. All three of these processes are vital in the synthesis and mobilization of immune factors. Thus, immunoincompetence is not a surprising outcome in deficiency. It is note-worthy that the T cell count falls in B_6 deficiency just as it does in AIDS (Table 1).

The clinical appearance of B_6 deficiency includes lesions on the skin and inside the mouth. Skin lesions are found on the face, neck, legs, and arms; mouth lesions are found on the tongue, lips, and on the surfaces of any walls. These lesions can serve as sites for fungal infections because the integrity of the skin is broken, and microbes have the opportunity to gain a foothold. Additionally, secretion of immune substances (immunoglobulin A [IgA]) at the skin and into the GI tract is low, resulting in depressed response to viral and bacterial challenges at these surfaces.

Fungal infection(s) further challenge the immune system, which is already weakened due to nutritional deficiency. In AIDS, fungal infections also appear on the skin and in the mouth, but they are not responsive to therapeutic doses of vitamin B_6 because deficiency is not the root cause. This is one of many examples in persons with AIDS (PWAs) where a disorder due to HIV resembles a nutritional deficiency. In this way, B_6 deficiency is like AIDS.

3. Vitamin B_{12}

Vitamin B_{12} (cobalamine) is required for nucleic acid (RNA, DNA) synthesis, a prerequisite for cell growth and multiplication. It is difficult to study the effect of cobalamine deficiency on immune status because the body stores are enormous; in humans, it could take as long as 5 years to deplete the stores. Nevertheless, B_{12} deficiency would impair the production of lymphocytes and antibodies. In this way, B_{12} deficiency produces a syndrome similar to AIDS.

4. Biotin

As with other B vitamins, the deficiency of biotin results in the loss of GI tract integrity and the appearance of spontaneous infections including *Candida* in the mouth cavity (Table 1). In this way, biotin deficiency is like AIDS.

5. Folic Acid

Folic acid plays a role in protein and nucleic acid metabolism throughout the body including the immune system. Therefore, in a deficiency of the vitamin, it is expected that the body's capacity to produce T lymphocytes and antibodies will be compromised (Table 1). Deficiency also results in the loss of GI tract integrity just as with some other vitamins (vitamins A, B_2, B_6, niacin). For both of these reasons, the body has increased susceptibility to microbial infection as it does in AIDS.

6. Niacin

Niacin deficiency results in a progressive illness characterized first by dermatitis and diarrhea (Table 1). The disease begins with failure to replace the old cells of the GI tract as they are sloughed, leaving a raw and exposed lining. It becomes irritated and inflamed starting with the mouth and moving down the throat, into the stomach and intestines. Due to irritation, the absorptive surface area of the small intestines is greatly reduced leading to diarrhea. The stomach may lose its capacity to secrete acid which allows microbes that come in with food to survive. These microbes can cause infection in the gut canal, and they may cross the gut wall since its integrity is lost, giving rise to infections inside the body. In these ways, niacin deficiency is like AIDS.

7. Pantothenic Acid

Pantothenic acid is involved in body metabolism at many points but not with protein. For this reason, it is not clear how it supports the immune system.

However, deficiency does lead to a loss of GI tract integrity and depressed lymphocyte count, as well as the capacity to produce new ones when challenged to do so (Table 1). In these two ways, pantothenic acid deficiency is like AIDS.

C. VITAMIN C

The role of vitamin C (ascorbic acid) is not clear except that it is present in relatively high levels in leukocytes circulating in the bloodstream. One type of leukocyte involved in immune function is the phagocyte that engulfs particles of invading bacteria and participates in the repair of wounds. Another type is the T lymphocyte. Ascorbic acid deficiency increases the susceptibility to infection, perhaps through reductions of the counts of both phagocytes and T lymphocytes (Table 1). In this way, vitamin C deficiency is like AIDS.

Nobel prize winner Linus Pauling popularized the intake of megadoses of ascorbic acid in order to fortify the body against infection and help it fight infections already underway. These claims remain controversial after many years. Scientists have not been able to validate or support supplementation with megadoses of ascorbic acid. In fact, research with humans indicates that intake in excess of need is simply excreted in the urine or not absorbed from the gut.

D. VITAMIN E

Tocopherols is the generic term given to the family of about eight chemically related compounds which have vitamin E activity. Tocopherols are located mostly in the membranes of all cells where they function as antioxidants. In this capacity, they protect polyunsaturated fatty acids in the membranes against the destructive attack by free radicals of oxygen.

The effects of tocopherol deficiency on immune function are indirect. In deficiency, membranes lose critical fatty acids, and the capacity of the cell to maintain its special mix of substances inside is lost. Consequently, cellular activity is lost, and the capacity to synthesize lymphocytes and antibodies is reduced (Table 1). In this way, tocopherol deficiency resembles AIDS.

E. MINERALS

It is difficult to study the role of minerals in immune function for several reasons. First, some are required in very tiny amounts, making it difficult to produce deficiency in experimental animals or to find humans with the deficiency syndrome. Second, minerals tend to interact with one another; a deficiency of one generally influences the activity or metabolism of another. Third, minerals serve as enzyme components that influence chemical reactions throughout the body, which makes it difficult to establish clearly their role in immune function.

Yet, research with minerals has shown links with the immune system for some, but not all. Often the clinical (visual) observation of infection implicates minerals, when diet and the results of selected laboratory tests are known. It is

TABLE 2
Changes in Immune Status with
Deficiencies of Selected Minerals

Mineral	Lymphocyte count	Antibody response
Cadmium	D	D
Chromium	D	—
Copper	—	PD
Iron	D	PD
Selenium	—	D
Zinc	D	D

Note: A = Atrophy, C = compromised, D = depression, PD = possible depression, N = normal, dash (—) = no data or no effect.

thought that the increased susceptibility to infections is the result of decreased lymphocyte production and/or possibly impaired antibody production (Table 2) among other changes. In these ways, mineral deficiencies are like AIDS.

Zinc is of special interest among the minerals because it gained notoriety early in the study of AIDS, before the proposition of a viral hypothesis. It was determined at the outset that homosexual (gay) men with AIDS had lower levels of circulating zinc than heterosexual males. In deficiency, lymphocyte function is depressed (Table 2). Therefore, it was initially thought that there might be a connection between zinc depletion and AIDS.

First, diet was ruled out. Then the search for an explanation of low zinc levels in PWAs led to the consideration of sexual activity. Gay men with AIDS often reported having sex much more frequently than heterosexual men. Hence, gay men had many more discharges of semen in any given period of time. Semen is known to be rich in zinc content; therefore, some investigators suggested that sexual "hyperactivity" might be responsible for AIDS. The demonstration that AIDS is caused by HIV ended this speculation.

III. PREDISPOSING FACTORS IN AIDS

A. SUSCEPTIBILITY TO HIV INFECTION

Despite the discovery of HIV as the causative agent in AIDS, some nutrition scientists have hypothesized that nutritional status still might play a key role. Underlying malnutrition might facilitate infection with the virus because the immune system is not optimally prepared to resist exposure. This hypothesis is interesting and perhaps controversial because it suggests that exposure to HIV does not necessarily mean that an individual will become infected. In other words, good nutrition might be prophylactic or protective against infection in the general sense that a condom protects against pregnancy for women or even HIV infection for men or women.

1. Quantity of Diet

Unfortunately, who gets infected by HIV may well be determined by diet and nutritional status. Diet is dependent on socioeconomic status as well as the abuse of drugs, which can divert money away from the purchase of food. Access to food (its availability and cost) is a major limitation on the economically disadvantaged "poor". By contrast, "rich" persons have more money to spend on food. This allows them to buy the food products they want without regard for cost, and they can purchase in the quantities desired. Therefore, those with adequate incomes have a greater nutritional opportunity than do the poor, and they may enjoy greater protection against infection as a result.

2. Nutrition Knowledge

Knowledge about diet and nutrition is another factor that may predispose the poor to HIV infection. It results from a blend of experiences with culture, religion, formal school learning, and exposure to television messages. It is hypothesized by many nutritionists that knowledge influences food selection behaviors, but this is still controversial. If behaviors can be driven by knowledge, then nutrition education could be used to help people obtain a high–quality, nutrient–rich diet.

The poor would be at a disadvantage, because of their limited opportunities, to build a knowledge base in comparison to wealthier individuals. The result is that the poor might select foods based on criteria other than nutritional value, and their diet would be of inferior quality. If this is true, then the poor would be more likely to be undernourished and might become infected with HIV more readily than better educated, well–fed persons.

B. PROGRESSION FROM HIV INFECTION TO AIDS

A second role of nutritional status is hypothesized to be in the speed with which AIDS develops after HIV infection. Good nutrition through a high–quality diet might slow it down while malnutrition due to a poor one might hasten its onset. Malnutrition is well known to compromise immune status (Sections I and II), and HIV adds to the problem by destroying certain components of the immune system, particularly T lymphocytes. Together, malnutrition and HIV infection increase the likelihood of opportunistic infections.

To add insult to injury, the opportunistic infections challenge the immune system, which is already weakened. This sets up a vicious cycle in which malnutrition, HIV infection, and opportunistic infections damage the immune system. Ultimately, no challenge can be sustained because the immune system is completely ravaged, and death results. Again, poor persons have less opportunity to achieve a high–quality diet in order to maximize nutritional status;

therefore, the time of onset for AIDS might be shorter for the poor than for well–fed persons.

IV. DIETARY RECOMMENDATIONS
FOR HEALTHY PERSONS

In order to understand dietary recommendations for persons with HIV and AIDS, it is helpful to know something about those designed for healthy persons. The U.S. Department of Agriculture (USDA) is the branch of the federal government that conducts research on the dietary behaviors and food preferences of Americans. This research helps to identify the foods that are important contributors of the various essential nutrients; for example, milk is a significant source of calcium in the American diet. Armed with this information, the USDA can make recommendations about what foods to include in the diet every day and how many servings should be eaten. You may be aware that the U.S. Department of Health and Human Services (US HHS) also makes recommendations concerning the diet, but its focus is different, concentrating instead on disease and disease prevention through the diet.

Two types of food guidance given to healthy Americans by the USDA include the "Dietary Guidelines for Americans"[18] and food guides. Both of these tools have been revised periodically because scientific knowledge and priorities for good health and eating preferences for Americans have changed over time. AIDS patients should make an effort to become aware of how food guidance does and does not fit with their needs when they first become infected. They should consider, too, the discussion of paradoxes between their needs and the priorities of healthy persons as set forth in the Dietary Guidelines (Section V.D).

A. UNITED STATES DIETARY GUIDELINES
The Dietary Guidelines are general recommendations for eating behaviors instead of rules specifying what foods to eat and how much to eat of them. The Dietary Guidelines are intended for healthy persons, not for individuals with disease such as those who have HIV infection or AIDS. There are seven guidelines as discussed below.

1. Eat a Variety of Foods
The first guideline is designed to ensure an adequate diet. No single food contains all required nutrients; however, by combining foods, it is very likely that healthy persons will get all of the nutrients that are needed. This first guideline is the basis for a "well–balanced" diet, a term which is often mentioned in discussions of nutrition and food. Balance implies that each of the many essential nutrients is consumed with none being present in levels that are too high or too low. This guideline is also a basic principle in diet planning, and it is applicable to persons infected with HIV and PWAs.

2. Maintain Healthy Weight

The purpose of this guideline is to focus attention on the relationship between disease and obesity. Being overweight increases the risk of becoming diabetic and having heart disease and hypertension. The solution is to achieve and maintain an "ideal" body weight. Your ideal body weight is usually determined by height, though this is not always a reliable criterion. The problem is that body builds differ among individuals, but this major factor cannot be considered for practical reasons.

There are other factors that come into play in the assessment of ideal body weight. For example, heavy muscularity has been a problem for bodybuilders in the Armed Services on numerous occasions. The bodybuilders find that they are classified as being "overweight" due to their high level of muscular development, yet they are not overfat. These cases are ironic, because athletes are supposed to be healthy but the Service weight guidelines indicate that they are not.

3. Fat and Cholesterol Intake

The third dietary guideline states, "Choose a diet low in fat, saturated fat, and cholesterol." This one is primarily designed to decrease the risk of coronary heart disease. It is not intended that any one food, such as red meat, should be excluded from the diet. Instead, the consumption of all animal products should be reduced across the board. This can be accomplished in a number of ways: (1) choose low–fat meats; (2) increase the intake of proteins such as dried beans and peas; (3) decrease egg consumption; (4) substitute polyunsaturated fats (vegetable margarines and shortenings) for sources high in saturated fats (butter, cream); (5) trim fat off meats; (6) avoid fried foods; and (7) be a label reader and avoid high–fat foods.

The relevance of this guideline to persons with HIV infection or AIDS is questionable. Heart disease develops over many years. Yet, the person with HIV or AIDS may not have a sufficient life span to benefit from the restriction of fats in the diet. It may be better not to limit their fat intake because the foods containing fat are most often animal products that are rich sources of protein, vitamins, and minerals. By encouraging the person with HIV or AIDS to eat various types of meats (beef, chicken, pork, and fish) and dairy products, his or her nutritional status could be maximized. This benefit may well outweigh any increase in the chance of getting heart disease.

4. Vitamins, Minerals, Starch, and Dietary Fiber

The fourth guideline states, "Choose a diet with plenty of vegetables, fruits, and grain products." Starch provides bulk to foods, and it helps to make a meal satisfying because it takes longer to digest than sugar. Additionally, carbohydrates are found in foods that tend to be good sources of nutrients while sugar is not. The best sources of complex carbohydrate in the typical American diet are grain products; fruits and vegetables are the next best source. Vitamins, minerals, and dietary fiber are all found in abundance in fruits, vegetables, and grain products.

Dietary fiber is a plant cell wall component that cannot be digested by human gut enzymes. There is no dietary fiber in animal products. Dietary fiber should not be confused with crude fiber, which is an outmoded concept. American diets tend to be low in dietary fiber. Increasing the intake of the dietary component reduces symptoms of constipation and diverticulosis. Additionally, it is possible that increasing the intake of dietary fiber may reduce the risk for colon cancer. For the PWA with diarrhea, it has been suggested that certain types of dietary fiber may be helpful in stopping or controlling the flow (Chapter 3).

5. Decrease Sugar Intake

"Use sugars only in moderation." The primary health problem with sugar is tooth decay; however, it also can have a negative impact on dietary quality. Foods rich in refined, "white" sugar are usually not good sources of essential nutrients. Therefore, when sugar–rich foods are eaten to excess, the nutritive value of the diet is diluted. It is recommended that a healthy diet should contain low amounts of refined sugar. Instead of refined sugars, it is suggested that naturally occurring sugars be consumed; these types of sugars are generally found in fruits and fruit juices.

The effects of refined sugar on the mouth and gum tissues are important concerns for persons with HIV or AIDS. Tooth decay and gingivitis are both caused by the formation of plaque on tooth or gum surfaces, respectively. Plaque is a film of mucus in which sugar–loving bacteria become trapped. In the process of consuming refined sugars, the bacteria produce acids, and these chemicals are responsible for the destruction of tooth surfaces or the irritation of gum tissue. Unfortunately, due to immune suppression, the plaque cannot be kept under the same control as it can be with healthy persons. For this reason, persons with HIV and AIDS might do well to reduce sugar intake and see their dentists frequently.

The issue of dietary quality is another matter. Sweet foods are more tempting to eat than others. Since it is often the case that PWAs need to consume food any way they can get it, it seems reasonable to feed them anything. However, when the patient's condition is stabilized, it is appropriate to move away from sugar–rich foods toward more nutritious ones (those containing more nutrients per calorie than sugar–rich foods).

6. Avoid Too Much Sodium

"Use salt and sodium only in moderation." Americans eat far more sodium than is needed to satisfy their requirement for this mineral nutrient. The problem with excess sodium intake is that it may be a risk factor for hypertension in susceptible individuals. The problem is that it is hard to know who is susceptible, but it is estimated that less than one in five Americans will become hypertensive. Therefore, it is prudent for all healthy persons to begin cutting back on the use of salt at the table and during food preparation. Additionally, it is a good idea to cut back on foods that have been heavily salted, including Chinese food (excess monosodium glutamate [MSG] contains sodium), chips, popcorn, nuts, brined pickles, cured meats (ham), and others.

7. Drink Alcoholic Beverages in Moderation

The argument for moderating alcohol intake is basically the same as for refined sugar. This source of calories does not contribute other nutrients, and hence it dilutes the nutritive intake of the diet. For some persons, alcohol serves as an appetite suppressant which further compounds the problem of reduced intake of essential nutrients.

B. DESIGN OF A FOOD GUIDE

A second major activity of the USDA is in providing food guidance. Over the years this has been done with a series of guides beginning with "Food Guide for Young Children" which was first published in 1916. The most successful has been the development of the familiar "basic four food groups", which have been modified several times after their release in the late 1950s.

A very interesting thing about USDA food guides is that they are not static. They change as dietary preferences and health priorities shift. They also have changed in complexity as the USDA and other agencies have wrestled with the need to balance the conflicting needs of simplicity and accuracy. However, it is surprising that the organization of foods in the guides changes as well. This indicates a continuing lack of consensus on some issues relating to the design of food guides; some of these issues are discussed below.

1. Variety

The well–balanced diet is based on the need for variety as previously introduced (Sections IV.A.1). Again, no single food contains all of the essential nutrients in the right amounts, and different kinds of foods will have to be eaten in order to satisfy the body's requirements (Section IV.A.1). These two facts are visually apparent in plots of leading nutrients by food group based on the eating habits of typical Americans (Table 3). The term "well–balanced diet" refers to the capacity of the diet to provide an optimal mix of essential nutrients to support the body, with all nutrients present at just the right levels. A food guide must be designed in such a way that its use results in a well–balanced diet.

2. Quantity

However the guide cannot stop there. It also recommends how much of each food or food group to consume. The reason is that the amount of nutrients found in the diet are related to the energy value of the foods containing them (Figure 1). This is important information for those with compromised immune systems because it means that a certain amount of food must be eaten to get

TABLE 3
Breakdown of the Traditional "Basic Four" Food Groups According to Contribution of 11 Nutrients and Energy to Typical American Diet

	Food Group			
Nutrient	Dairy products	Meat and alternates	Grain products	Fruits and vegetables
Energy		X	X	
Protein		X		
Vitamin A				X
Vitamin C				X
Vitamin B_1		X	X	
Vitamin B_2	X	X	X	
Vitamin B_6		X		X
Niacin		X	X	
Calcium	X		X	
Iron		X	X	
Magnesium		X	X	X
Phosphorus	X	X	X	

Note: The leading source(s) of each nutrient has (have) been identified with an "X" to indicate a contribution equal to or greater than 20% of total daily intake where the cutoff value is high and arbitrary. (Data from *1977–1978 Nationwide Food Consumption Survey,* U.S. Department of Agriculture, Washington, D.C.)

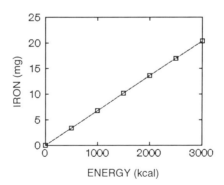

FIGURE 1. Relationship between dietary energy content and iron intake; as caloric intake increases, so does iron intake at a rate of about 6.8 mg/1000 kcal.[8]

all the nutrients needed to help fight HIV infection and other possible opportunistic infections (Section III.B). It will be difficult for an anorexic to eat enough food to get the necessary nutrients. That is why infected persons who are anorexic must make every effort to eat even if it seems like work (Section V.A.5.c).

3. Food Groups

A basic concept of a food guide is that foods can be grouped together by nutritive contents (Table 3). The original basic four food groups were famous for: (1) meat and alternates; (2) dairy products; (3) fruits and vegetables; and (4) grain products. Foods in each of these four groups were like one another in nutritive value in most cases.

Sometimes foods within a group differed by origin. For example, the meat and alternates group contained eggs and beef. These two foods do not come from the same animal, but they were placed in the same group because they are both good sources of protein. On the other hand, cheese, which is a good source of protein, was put in with dairy products because users felt all products from a cow should be together.

Another interesting example of the organization of foods into groups happened in 1979 with the addition of a fifth group to the famous four. This group consisted of fats and sweets, and the basis of their being grouped together was that all of the foods were poor sources of essential nutrients.

a. *1977–1978 Nationwide Food Consumption Survey*

The 1977–1978 Nationwide Food Consumption Survey (77–78 NFCS)[8] was sponsored by the USDA in order to determine what foods provided specific nutrients to Americans. This type of dietary survey addresses cultural food preferences, as well as the issues surrounding access to food (for example, availability and cost). The value of the information is in learning which foods people will and will not eat. Remember that a food may be a rich source of a given nutrient, but if it is not eaten, then it is of no value. One way to address this problem is to consider individual food likes and dislikes in planning the guide so that recommendations will be followed.

A discussion of food groups and the 77–78 NFCS follows.[8] In this discussion, food groups are recognized as "leading" sources of nutrients. Applied here, this term means that the food group provided 20% or more of total intake for typical Americans. This is an arbitrary and high cutoff value. Its usefulness is in distinquishing from among the four groups which ones are and are not the important or major sources for any given nutrient relative to the foods that Americans actually eat.

b. *Meat and Alternates Group*

The meat and meat alternates group includes all muscle foods (beef, poultry, fish, and pork), eggs, and legumes (any seed that comes in a pod, including peanuts and peanut butter). This group is noted as a leading source of 7 of the 11 vitamins and minerals in the typical American diet reported in the 77–78 NFCS.[8] These nutrients are protein; vitamins B_1 (thiamin), B_2 (riboflavin), and B_6 (pyridoxine); iron; magnesium; and phosphorus (Table 3). Additionally, meat and meat alternatives are a leading source of energy due to their high fat content.

There is often confusion as to what foods are members of this group. The rule is that any food containing a large amount of protein is a member. The confusion lies in the mixing together of foods of dissimilar origins in this group. "Meat" is taken to mean all foods that serve as a contractile muscle in an animal. This means that beef, pork, fish, and poultry all belong to the group. Yet, some people have the idea that only beef is meat because it is red while the others are white. However, color is not the criterion for inclusion; the criterion is protein content.

Meat is the usual standard against which other sources of dietary protein are compared. If the comparison of a food with meat is favorable with regard to its contribution of protein to the diet, then it is categorized as a meat alternate and included in the group; however, this is a confusing matter for many people, especially children. For example, cheese has sometimes been categorized as a meat alternate. Cheese is a concentrated form of milk, and as such it is a good source of protein. The problem is that cheese originates from a cow, and many people cannot understand why it is not located in the dairy products group.

Possibly due to this confusion, the most recent version of USDA dietary planning advice—"The Food Guide Pyramid"[17]—puts cheese in with other dairy products (milk, yogurt). This reflects a new approach that food guidance systems should be designed with foods of similar origin grouped together in order to reduce confusion. This practice negates the basic premise of traditional food guides that foods can by grouped by nutritive value.

c. Dairy Products Group

The 77–78 NFCS included all dairy products in this category; cheeses were lumped with fluid milk and yogurt.[8] The information collected revealed that the role of dairy products in the typical American diet was to provide three vitamins and minerals: vitamins B_2 (riboflavin), calcium, and phosphorus (Table 3).

d. Grain Products Group

The grain products group is noted as a leading source of 6 of the 11 vitamins and minerals in the typical American diet reported in the 77–78 NFCS.[8] These nutrients are vitamins B_1 (thiamin) and B_2 (riboflavin), calcium, iron, magnesium, and phosphorus (Table 3). Additionally, grain products are a leading source of energy due to their complex carbohydrate content. The fact that grain products are leading sources of thiamin, riboflavin, niacin, and iron is due to the enrichment (addition of nutrients) of virtually all flour produced for distribution and sale in the United States.

e. Fruits and Vegetables Group

The fruits and vegetables group is noted as a leading source of 4 of the 11 vitamins and minerals in the typical American diet reported in the 77–78 NFCS.[8] These nutrients are vitamins A (retinol), C (ascorbic acid), B_6 (pyridoxine), and magnesium (Table 3).

f. Fats and Sweets Group

Sweet–tasting foods that are mostly composed of sugar and very high–fat foods are classified by the USDA as members of the "fats and sweets" food group. These foods are energy rich, even though typical Americans did not eat enough in the 1970s for them to be leading sources of calories. However, if PWAs emphasized fats and sweets in their diets to help fight anorexia, then this food group could well contribute significantly to energy intake (Section V.A.5).

Unfortunately, fats and sweets are not good sources of essential nutrients. They were not leading sources of any of the 11 reported in the 77–78 NFCS.[8] In fact, the decision to include fats and sweets into one group was made on the basis of their *lack* of nutrient content, the so–called "empty calorie" foods.

4. Simplicity

Simply stated, if a food guide is overly complicated, then it will not be used because no one can remember how to use it. A good food guide makes use of instructional principles that facilitate its use by children, teenagers, and adults. This often is a difficult proposition because children and adults do not solve problems (i.e., think) in the same way. Additionally, it is difficult to design a guide for simplicity when there is a simultaneous need for accuracy. As the degree of accuracy increases, so does the level of complexity.

Ironically, the simplicity of popular guides such as the familiar basic four is a turnoff to some adults who feel that they need more sophisticated, adult–oriented dietary advice. These persons have a legitimate complaint in expressing their desire for details and explanations behind the recommendations. However, it is important to remember that a good food guide is firmly grounded in food and nutrition science whether or not it is simply stated. Food guides do not have to be complicated to work.

C. USDA FOOD GUIDES
1. Food Guide for Young Children

This first guide was called "Food Guide for Young Children",[16] and it featured five food groups. The groups were (1) vegetables and fruits; (2) milk, eggs, cheese, "flesh" foods, fish, and legumes; (3) cereals and other starchy foods; (4) sweets; and (5) fats. The grouping of foods was made on the basis of "their functions in the body..." (i.e., roles as they were understood at the time).

A number of features about the guide are notable. The grouping together of eggs, milk, cheese, beans, peas, and meat was made because of their protein content. Later guides put dairy products into a different group in recognition of their calcium content and/or source of origin (i.e., like is grouped according to like).

Although sugar and starchy foods were both known to be rich sources of carbohydrates, they were put into different groups apparently on the basis of flavor. Starchy foods are mild or bland, while sugar is sweet. Sugar has always been highly prized as a sweetening agent that serves to heighten interest in foods (Section V.A.5.b). In any event, these foods were probably not grouped differently on the basis of vitamin and mineral content because nutrition science and organic chemistry had not progressed to make that distinction possible.

Fat–rich foods were also placed in an independent group based on their energy value and "enrichment" of the diet (probably a reference to the contribution of flavor and texture to food and/or the "staying power" of meals). The only group that appears to be intuitively obvious is the one for fruits and vegetables.

"Food Guide for Young Children" was designed before nutrition science began to solve the mysteries of metabolism, deficiency diseases, and the nature of essential nutrients. For example, the B–complex factor was thought to be essential in the diet of man, but the individual vitamins were not known. In this regard, the food guide served a valuable role by helping people to plan nutritious diets even though it was not known how such diets worked.

2. Food for Fitness—A Daily Food Guide

The "Daily Food Guide", commonly known as the "basic four" or "four food groups", was unveiled in 1958[15] and revised several times afterward. This guide was a simplification of an earlier effort by USDA (1946) in which seven food groups were presented. The "Daily Food Guide" was enormously popular, perhaps because of its simplicity. Unlike "Food for Young Children", the "Daily Food Guide" did not formally recognize a group of foods as fats and/ or sweets. The reason was that these foods did not make significant contributions of essential nutrients to the diet; their energy value was ignored. Hence, a fats and sweets group would be of limited value from the perspective of nutrition education focused on foods as sources of essential nutrients, especially in light of the desire to keep the guide as simple as practical.

Another difference between these two early USDA guides was the treatment of dairy products. In the "Daily Food Guide", dairy products were removed from the protein–rich group of meat and alternates; they were put into a group of their own in order to recognize them as important sources of calcium.

Finally, the "Daily Food Guide" was designed to provide 1200 kcal and 80% of the 1953 Recommended Dietary Allowances (RDA) for eight vitamins and minerals. It was expected that individuals would eat more food than recommended in order to meet energy needs, and from this extra food would come the balance of nutrients needed for good health.

3. Hassle–Free Guide

The "Hassle–Free" guide was published in 1979; it was the fourth revision of the "Daily Food Guide" notable in that a fifth group of fats, sweets, and alcohol was formally added. This made the familiar basic four into the basic five, which did not seem to please anyone due to its increased complexity. The addition of the fifth group was made in response to the growing public

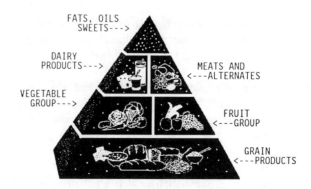

FIGURE 2. The Food Guide Pyramid is the latest food guide from the U.S. Department of Agriculture;[17] it is designed to visually indicate how much emphasis to place on each food group in the diet according to the dedicated area of the pyramid where the tip (smallest area) gets the least emphasis and the base (largest area) gets the most: fats and sweets group — use sparingly; dairy products — 2–3 servings per day; meat and alternates — 2–3 servings; fruits — 2–4 servings; vegetables — 3–5 servings; and grain products — 6–11 servings.

awareness of possible health risks associated with consumption of fats and sweets that could no longer be ignored.

4. Food Guide Pyramid

The "Food Guide Pyramid" was developed and supported by the joint efforts of the USDA and the US HHS (Figure 2): "It goes beyond the 'basic four food groups' to help you put the 'Dietary Guidelines' into action."[17] As with all USDA food guides, the pyramid is based on research into the eating habits of Americans to determine which particular foods are eaten and which are not. However, it is different because it has recommendations incorporated into its design that may reduce the risk of certain diseases, including coronary heart disease, hypertension, obesity, diabetes, alcoholism, tooth decay, and cancer.

To accomplish its goal to lower the risk of some diseases, the pyramid was designed to decrease dietary cholesterol, total fat, saturated fat, sugar, sodium, and alcohol. The emphasis on decreasing fat intake is strongest because it is most clear that the typical American diet is high in fat, and there could be some relationships between fat intake and disease. Nutrients that are emphasized by the pyramid include dietary fiber, vitamins, minerals, and complex carbohydrates (starch).

The "Food Guide Pyramid" categorizes foods into six major food groups (Figure 2). Each of the five food groups on the lower levels of the pyramid provides some, but not all, required nutrients.

The tip of the pyramid shows fats, oils, and sweets. These are foods such as salad dressings and oils, cream, butter, margarine, sugars, soft drinks, candies, and sweet desserts. These foods are good sources of energy.

The second level down on the pyramid is for protein–rich foods, mostly of animal origin. The two groups represented are the meat and alternates and dairy products. Since these foods tend to be high in fat content, the number of servings recommended is only two or three per day of each group.

The third level down is for the fruit and vegetable groups. It is recommended that three to five servings from the vegetable group be consumed each day. Two to four servings of fruit are also recommended each day. The base of the pyramid includes foods from the grain products group, for which the recommended number of servings is 6 to 11 per day.

One important difference between the basic four system and the pyramid is that the former specified fewer servings. It was up to the consumer to select foods to satisfy energy needs. These foods might or might not be rich sources of nutrients. By comparison, the pyramid provides guidance for a variable number of servings for each group. This suggests the manner in which the diet can be scaled up or down in energy content with high–quality foods.

V. DIETARY RECOMMENDATIONS FOR PERSONS INFECTED WITH HIV

Dietary recommendations made by health care professionals for persons infected with HIV and AIDS are based on nutritional objectives, each of which is designed to help the immune system do its job. However, these objectives often require formal reasoning skills for comprehension. Not only does this make them seem remote and unfriendly, but it also makes them subject to misinterpretation when the user is not familiar with the scientific jargon. The solution is to connect objectives to action–oriented statements for dietary behaviors that are given in plain language.

A. ENERGY INTAKE
1. Definition of Energy

Energy is not a nutrient. Instead, it is "the power to do work" that is contained in certain food components including carbohydrates, fats, protein, and alcohol. The energy in these nutrients is released during breakdown that can occur in any cells of the body including those that make immune factors such as T lymphocytes and antibodies. The energy power of foods is commonly expressed in terms of calories.

Today, the term calorie is seldom used by professionals in speaking or writing activities. It fell out of favor many years ago because a little calorie, spelled with a lower case "c", is not a useful expression of food energy; it is too small. The use of a large calorie, spelled with an upper case "C", was fashionable for writing purposes, but it could not be used in speech because it could never be determined whether a large or small calorie was meant by the speaker. Modern nutritionists use the metric system; and the term to express the energy value of food is "kilocalorie", where this unit represents 1000 small calories or a single large Calorie. Today, you will find the kilocalorie (kcal) notation on all nutrition labels in the United States.

TABLE 4
The Relationship Between
Energy Intake and Output
on Balance and Body Weight

Balance	Relationship[a]	Body weight
Positive	Intake > output	Gain
Negative	Intake < output	Loss
Zero	Intake = output	Constant

[a] (>) indicates "greater than"; (<) indicates "less than"; (=) indicates equality.

2. Energy Balance

Energy balance is an idea or concept relating the amount of energy you consume in food to that which is expended (Table 4). There are a variety of factors that determine energy expenditure including age, sex, body size, climate (i.e., heat production), and physical activity (i.e., sleep, waking rest, and exercise—light, moderate, and heavy). If more energy is taken in than is expended, then balance is positive (+) and body weight is gained. When intake is less than output, then balance is negative (–) and weight is lost over time. Zero balance (0) occurs when intake equals output, and there is no change in weight over time.

3. HIV, AIDS, and Body Weight Control

Infected persons, especially those with AIDS, should make every effort to be in positive or zero energy balance. If they are in negative balance, then there is a practical risk of malnutrition, which could compromise an immune function already damaged by the virus. This may hasten the onset of AIDS as well as death (Section III.B). Another important reason for maintaining energy balance is that body weight is a predictor of the incidence of disease and death. In other words, as your body weight falls toward a critical level, you will be much more likely to get opportunistic infections and cancers, and your chances of dying increase (Section V.A.5 and Chapter 2).

Objective No. 1:   *Maintain/achieve zero or positive energy balance.*

Recommendation No. 1: *Maintain body weight or make small gains.*

4. Demands of the Immune System

The most important nutritional objective concerns the need of the immune system for energy (Section II.B.1). To understand this need, it is convenient to compare the immune system to a small "army" where immune factors serve as the "soldiers". There is a cost to build and maintain each soldier of the army, and that cost involves energy.

In the healthy individual, a small army is kept on active duty at all times. This enables the body to do battle against invading microbes at a moment's notice. However, the army is small and it cannot win a "war" unless more soldiers can be called into action quickly. Energy is required to make new soldiers or immune factors, and hence a microbial challenge puts a heavy demand on the body's resources for energy.

It might be argued that it would be good to maintain a large army all the time. This way it would not be necessary to wait for new soldiers to be made in response to a microbial challenge; however, the maintenance of a large army would be very wasteful of energy resources during "peace time", and therefore it is not done.

When energy is in short supply, the process of making new soldiers for the army grinds to a halt just the way a car stops running when the gas tank is empty. Consequently, the microbial invaders go unchecked, and an infection will probably result. Thus, a lack of energy jeopardizes the ability of the army to protect the body.

5. Fighting Anorexia

Research with PWAs has demonstrated that there is a minimum amount of body cell mass (BCM) required for survival, and the timing of death is related to its depletion (Chapter 2). Ironically, some persons with HIV infection and even AIDS might attempt to deliberately lose weight for the sake of appearance. This should not be attempted because it amounts to voluntary starvation. Potential malnutrition and compromised immune function may increase the risk of disease complications with AIDS as well as the risk of death (Section III.B).

In undeveloped countries, negative energy balance and body weight loss are likely due to the lack of food. The effects of starvation are visually apparent. This is why AIDS is known as the "slim" disease in some undeveloped countries including those in central Africa. The physical appearance of PWAs shows marked loss of body weight as fat tissue (adipose) and skeletal muscle (Chapter 2).

By contrast, a negative energy balance in individuals living in industrialized nations is more likely to be due to anorexia (lack of desire to eat what is available), nausea induced by drugs (Chapter 5), or physiological changes in the GI tract due to lesions, infection, or therapy (Chapters 3 and 4). It is critical to be able to recognize anorexia and to take appropriate action to correct it. Anorexia, which results in a negative energy balance and weight loss, is a loss

TABLE 5
Procedure for Precise Monitoring of Body Weight

1. Wake up from night's sleep
2. Do not eat or drink anything
3. Urinate and have bowel movement, if needed
4. Take off clothing
5. Carefully weigh on scales (hospital-type preferred)
6. Record and plot bodyweight; look for a trend (up, down, or steady) in weight over several days and adjust food intake according to desired weight or trend

of the desire to eat or to engage in feeding behaviors; it can be caused by a multitude of factors, especially drugs prescribed for various illnesses that are common in persons with HIV infection. There are at least two important problems with restricted food intake. One of these is malnutrition, which can hasten the onset of AIDS and death (Section III.B). The other is the loss of body cell mass to a critical level resulting in death (Chapter 1, Section V.A.3 and Chapter 2).

Objective No. 2:   *Recognize anorexia.*

Recommendation No. 2:   *Weigh yourself regularly.*

---

a. Watching Your Weight

It is easy to recognize anorexia by monitoring an individual's body weight every day (Table 5). The following weighing procedure takes only a few minutes each day to complete and will become routine very quickly. In order to produce the desired results, the procedure must be followed carefully. To help the patient understand and appreciate the procedure, each step is explained in the analysis that follows.

Step 1. Body weight is best measured on awakening from the night's sleep.

Step 2. Do not eat or drink anything just before weighing. Food and beverages are heavy. For example, one cup of water weighs about 234 grams (1/2 pound). On a good set of hospital scales, you can achieve measurements indicating changes of as little as 100 grams (1/4 pound). Therefore, drinking just one cup of fluid will counteract any sensitivity you can achieve with your scale and greatly reduce the value of the weigh–in process.

Step 3. Urine and feces also add weight, but it is not a reflection of body tissues. Therefore, it is important to void (urinate) and defecate (as necessary) before weighing in; most people void in the morning when they rise. Urine is comprised mostly of water; not surprisingly, one cup of urine weighs about 234 grams (1/2 pound). A bowel movement can have a large impact on body weight measurement because a large stool can weigh 454 to 908 grams (1 to 2 pounds). Clearly, if you fail to void or defecate (as necessary), then you will get a misleading reading on the scale.

Step 4. Weigh naked or in the same clothing day after day. Just as food, beverages, urine, and feces do, clothing adds weight to your body. Consider these examples of the weight of selected pieces of clothing: socks, T–shirt, and briefs—200 grams (0.4 pounds); flannel shirt—500 grams (1.1. pounds); western cut jeans—900 grams (2.0 pounds); cowboy boots—1600 grams (3.5 pounds); motorcycle boots—2100 grams (4.6 pounds); motorcycle jacket—2300 grams (5.1 pounds).

If you must wear clothing during weigh–in, then wear the exact same pieces every time. This practice will cancel out its effect on your weight because the exact same value for the clothing will be added to your true weight every time you weigh in. This will still permit you to monitor trends in your weight (see Step 7). However, if you want to determine your true weight, then you will have to do without clothing at weigh–in.

Step 5. Use your scales with care, and keep them in a protected location. Your scales should be dedicated for your use alone; do not allow other persons to weigh on them. The reason for these rules is to keep your scales working the same way time after time, with good sensitivity, for as long as you own them.

There are three important considerations when purchasing a set of scales. *Cost* can be a deciding factor. It is important, however, to recognize that all scales are not created equal; cost may be one factor reflecting quality. Quality is the capacity to make *precision* measurements, giving consistent weights for the same person, day after day. Additionally, precision is the capacity to measure or detect a change in body weight. Sensitive scales for measuring the body weight of adults can detect changes of as little as 100 grams (about 1/4 pound). It is not practical to measure smaller changes because there is some "background noise" (small, unexplained changes from day to day in body weight, which would otherwise be amplified, demanding attention that is not deserved). In addition to precision, *accuracy* is another important quality attribute of weighing scales. It is the ability to measure true or actual weight. Some people think that knowing the true weight is unimportant. In their viewpoint, it is more important that the scales are precise, weighing in the same manner each day. In so doing, trends will emerge. From these trends, it is possible to assess whether your bodyweight is increasing, decreasing, or staying the same over days.

There are generally two kinds of scales. One is the familiar bathroom scale, which is low in cost but not known for its precision. At the top end are the hospital scales seen at doctors' offices (Figure 3). The precision of these scales is often very good, but they are expensive (around $150 to $200). If body weight control is to be seriously pursued, then the hospital scales would be the better choice for purchase.

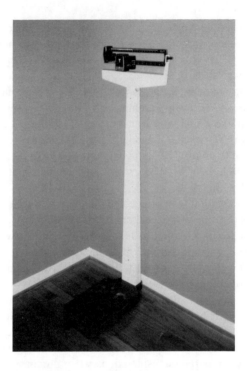

FIGURE 3. Physician's examining scale for weighing adults, commonly known as hospital scales or balance beam scales (*Health-o-meter, Continental Scale Corp.; Bridgeview, Illinois*).

Step 6. Plot data each day. This will help you to see any trend or direction in the data. Look for trends over several days or longer. Short–term, day–to–day fluctuations are often attributable to background "noise". They may not reflect real or actual trends in weight to which you should pay attention. These short–term changes often reflect metabolic or dietary phenomenon including net gain ("bloating") or loss (dehydration) of water, buildup of fecal material due to irregular bowel function, or changes in diet composition as a result of an increase or decrease in dietary fiber intake.

Figure 4 shows a plot of body weight data with a trend line (linear regression) for a PWA. During this period, he did not intentionally try to lose weight; however, the trend of the plotted data indicates that weight decreased by 1.5 kilograms (3.4 pounds) over the 30–day study period or about 0.8 lb/week. Thus, he was in negative energy balance during the recording period (Section V.A.2). The rate of loss is not fast relative to the maximum of 1.0 kilogram (2.0 pounds) per week recommended for healthy persons by the American Dietetic Association; however, it may be a fast rate for PWAs. In fact, no weight loss may be acceptable for PWAs in light of evidence linking weight loss with the increased risks for disease and death (Section III.B).

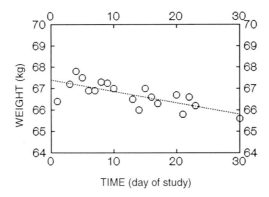

FIGURE 4. Body weight vs. time for a sedentary male person with AIDS who was unaware of negative energy balance.

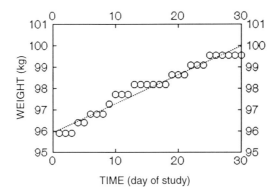

FIGURE 5. Body weight vs. time for a healthy male athlete training with weights to increase muscle size; energy intake was deliberately high to result in positive balance.

Due to noise in the data, the PWA's weight bounces around the trend line from day to day, as can be seen in the plot (Figure 4). Again, this noise problem points to the need to consider the data over time rather than on a day–by–day basis.

An uninfected, 26–year–old male fitness instructor agreed to record his weight and share it for comparison purposes (Figure 5). This former athlete was "bulking up", striving for maximum muscle gains with a minimum addition of fat by training heavily with weights and increasing caloric intake at the same time to cause weight gain (positive energy balance). He made an increase of 3.9 kilograms (8.6 pounds) over the 30–day study period or 2.0 pounds per week. This rapid increase in body weight is reflected in the trend line for the plotted data (Figure 5).

Note how data points are "stair stepped" on the plot. The subject rounded daily weight values to the nearest whole pound instead of to the nearest 1/4 pound, the ideal level of sensitivity. Because of rounding, some sensitivity in the data was removed; consequently, noise was decreased. While the bodybuilder's plot (Figure 5) is cleaner, the PWA's is more realistic (Figure 4).

b. Coaxing Oneself to Eat

To combat anorexia and negative energy balance, it is necessary to identify and select foods for which you have a personal preference when possible. You already know which foods are your favorites, but you do not want to serve such a limited diet because it quickly will become tiresome. Therefore, it is necessary to add other foods to round out your menu. This can easily be done by considering several characteristics of foods. First, there is visual appearance, including surface texture and color. After all, foods that do not pass visual inspection on the plate may not make it to the mouth. The second critical characteristic of foods is smell or aroma; foods that do not have a pleasing aroma also may not make it to the mouth. Of course, the mouth is the center of taste sensations, and taste is crucial to the acceptance of any food. Another phenomenon going on in the mouth during the intake of food is the brain's assessment of how that food feels against the mouth walls—hot or cold, soft or hard, and so on; all this information influences the brain's perception of acceptability.

Objective No. 3:	*Address anorexia.*
Recommendation No. 3:	*Select food based on personal preferences or favorites.*

To make the point that foods can be very different in desirability, consider the following comparison. Imagine a thick, buttered slice of homemade bread just out of the oven; it smells terrific and has very mild traces of sweet and salt tastes; the crumb is soft and pretty white contrasting with a golden crust all the way around the slice. Now imagine a dish of sauerkraut with its characteristic gray–white color, tough strands of fine–sliced cabbage, strong tastes of acid (sour) and salt, and pungent vinegar smell.

In your mind, compare what it would be like to eat the bread vs. the sauerkraut. Is it fair to say that eating strongly flavored sauerkraut is a more intense experience than the bread? Is it not true that you have to learn to like sauerkraut over time while bread is more readily accepted and enjoyed due to its mild and pleasing combination of sensory attributes? Some believe that sick persons prefer mildly flavored foods over strong ones because the strong ones can elicit unpleasant sensations such as nausea and/or vomiting. Again, the point is that the sensory experiences of food are important to consider when PWAs select food for themselves.

Of the four basic tastes, it is well known through sensory evaluation experiments that people respond more favorably to the sweet sensation than bitter, salt, or sour. Therefore, it makes sense to consider sweet foods in the battle against anorexia; sweet foods are most likely to be tolerated. Some sweet, "fun" foods are ice cream, coffee cake, candy, cookies, donuts, juices, milk shakes, sugar–sweetened soft drinks, and hot and cold breakfast cereals.

Notwithstanding the good acceptance of sweet foods, fun foods are not always sweet. Protein–rich foods can also be fun to eat, particularly when they are identified with an age group or lifestyle. For example, hamburgers and pizza are very popular with teenagers and young adults. In any event, protein–rich foods in general are highly valued by Americans. These foods are a part of the culture, they taste good, and they are available at practical cost. All of these factors help to ensure that certain nutrients will be present in the diet including high–quality protein, vitamins, and minerals. Of special note is the love affair which Americans have with beef steak—it is an excellent source of protein, vitamins, and minerals (Table 3).

Another category of fun food is that which provides an abundance of calories from fat. This nutrient has more than twice as many calories per gram weight (fat = 9 kilocalories per gram) than protein (4) or carbohydrate (4), thus fat–rich foods really pack an energy punch. Familiar fat–rich foods include potato chips and other chip snacks, french fried potatoes, regular salad dressings, bacon, and all types of salad oil, vegetable shortening, butter, and margarine. It is commonly recommended that fatty foods be consumed by PWAs in order to boost caloric intakes; however, there is a need to be somewhat cautious because fat digestion and absorption in the small intestine is sometimes impaired (Chapter 3). The inability to digest and absorb fat is evidenced by the excretion of cream–colored, fatty stools (i.e., steatorrhea).

Admittedly, fun foods are not always the best sources of important nutrients such as protein, vitamins, and minerals. When compared with the other four food groups (Section IV.B.3.e), fats and sweets are not leading sources of essential nutrients listed. However, they are not devoid of nutritional value if energy content is considered, and energy is a prime concern for the hospitalized PWA. Besides the fact that fat and/or sweet fun foods are enjoyable, they generally do not produce sugar intolerance (Chapter 3) or aggravate diarrhea because of their low dietary fiber content (Chapter 3).

c. Eating as a Job

It is one thing to recommend fun foods, but that does not mean that it will always be fun to eat them. The process can still be difficult because feelings of nausea, diarrhea, and other complications of AIDS and drug treatment can wipe out any desire to eat.

Under this circumstance, it will be necessary for the patient to adopt the attitude that he or she has a job to do, a responsibility to devote a certain amount of time and effort each day just to eating food. More specifically, the consumption of a certain amount of food each day should be targeted, even if it takes a long time. Optimally, the targeted amount of food will provide enough energy to maintain body weight.

B. PROTEIN INTAKE

Protein follows energy in importance for the immune system. Immune factors are largely built from components of protein. The typical American diet contains an abundance of protein because protein–rich foods are a part of the culture, they are available and affordable, and the taste is desirable. Typical Americans consume more than the RDA for protein. There appears to be nothing wrong with this excess; the RDA was not intended to be used as a basis for lowering habitual intakes. For example, the RDA for protein is about 0.4 grams per pound of body weight, but most American males consume about 150% RDA or 0.6 grams per pound. To compare and contrast, athletes generally consume much higher levels—from 1.0 gram per pound up to 6.0 (or more).

The RDA was designed to serve as a safe, lower level of intake that would prevent disease and promote good health; it was not formulated for persons who are sick. Illness represents a significant nutritional challenge for which protein needs are elevated (the increased need for energy has been discussed above in Section V.A.4). The enhanced requirement for protein is the result of metabolic activities that prepare the body to fight infection. HIV is an especially difficult challenge because it is chronic in nature, and the body is continually stimulated to make an immune response. This tends to divert protein intake and deplete tissue protein reserves, especially skeletal muscle (Chapter 2).

There is no guideline defining an optimal level of dietary protein for persons infected with HIV or the opportunistic infections of AIDS, but it seems reasonable to regard the RDA as a "floor" level (i.e., a minimum acceptable target). One possible strategy is to use the RDA as a benchmark, increasing it to a level that can be practically achieved. For example, since typical American males routinely consume roughly 150% RDA for protein, this level of intake might be practical for the PWA, also.

Objective No. 4:   *Achieve a generous protein intake.*

Recommendation No. 4:   *Eat a variety of foods consistent
                              with the typical American diet.*

A still higher protein intake level might be helpful, but may not be practical because it would involve deliberate efforts to incorporate protein–rich foods in the diet to the exclusion of other, more familiar foods and the grocery bill could be higher. For example, the efforts of athletes to achieve very high protein diets are well known: bodybuilders have reported intakes of 400 to 600% RDA. There is no solid evidence, however, to indicate that any given, high level of protein intake is protective against muscle wasting and the increased demands of the overstimulated immune system.

As a general rule, low protein intakes are not due to poor food choice behavior or lack of access (availability and affordability). Instead, the chief obstacle among PWAs is more likely to be anorexia. It is important to recognize that anorexia is not specifically directed at protein–rich foods to the exclusion of others. The disorder is a generalized loss of desire to eat food or to engage in behaviors associated with eating. When anorexia is identified and addressed, it is possible that normal eating behaviors will return and a variety of foods will be consumed in the manner of typical Americans. In this variety will come the usual, plentiful supply of protein Americans enjoy.

C. VITAMIN AND MINERAL INTAKE

The importance of selected vitamins and minerals for immune function has been discussed (Section II). Additionally, the case for variety in food choices to achieve the proper intake of these essential nutrients has also been presented (Sections IV.A.1 and IV.B.1). The appropriate use of dietary supplements ("pill" form) to add vitamins and minerals into the diet will be discussed (Section V.E). For HIV–infected persons, it seems appropriate to plan a well–balanced diet and to take a dietary supplement.

Objective No. 5:	*Achieve a generous intake of vitamins and minerals from foods.*
Recommendation No. 5:	*Eat a variety of foods consistent with the typical American diet, and eat generous amounts of these foods.*

Data from the 77–78 NFCS can be used to determine which food groups are leading sources of various essential nutrients (Sections IV.B.3.a–e); this information has also been tabulated for visual inspection (Table 3). In order to obtain all of the essential nutrients from food sources, it is necessary to combine the food groups and to consume practical amounts or numbers of servings from each on a daily basis.

Healthy persons can look to the RDA for guidance in appropriate vitamin and mineral intakes. Again, the RDAs were designed to serve as safe, lower levels of intake that prevent disease and promote good health. They were not formulated for persons who are sick, including those with the HIV infection.

The enhanced requirement for vitamins and minerals is the result of metabolic activities that prepare the body to fight infection. HIV is an especially difficult challenge because it is chronic in nature. The body is continually stimulated to make an immune response, and this tends to deplete vitamin and mineral stores.

Intakes of vitamin and minerals probably should exceed the RDA for PWA, preferably through food sources. However, it is recognized that people do not always "eat right". Some "insurance" can be obtained by taking a multivitamin and mineral supplement (Section V.E). The emphasis on obtaining vitamins and minerals from food sources instead of supplements or "pills" is made because naturally occurring vitamins and minerals can be more likely to be absorbed into the body; this is particularly true for minerals (Section V.E).

Another important reason for eating food sources of vitamins and minerals is that scientists do not know about all of the dietary factors that contribute to good nutrition. There may be as yet unidentified essential nutrients present in foods. Then again, nutrients appear in foods in a "natural", balanced relationship. Some nutritionists believe that this relationship might be important in vitamin and mineral absorption and utilization in the body.

D. PARADOX WITH THE DIETARY GUIDELINES

The third edition of "Dietary Guidelines for Americans"[18] de–emphasizes fun foods which provide "empty calories" from refined sugar and fat. The term empty calories implies that fun foods are poor sources of protein, vitamins, and minerals, but they are good sources of energy. This creates two problems. First, these foods are limited in their capacity to improve the nutritional status of the body as a whole. Second, they cannot even provide the essential vitamins and minerals to be used in their own metabolism; therefore, they put a drain on the body's supplies of vitamins and minerals.

While empty calorie foods can be poor sources of protein, vitamins, and minerals, they tend to be rich sources of saturated fat, cholesterol, and sugar. It is widely believed that the high–fat diet of Americans, with its high content of saturated fat and cholesterol, is related to the long–term development of chronic illnesses including heart disease and certain cancers. High sugar intake is clearly linked to tooth decay. Additionally, a high–sugar, high–fat diet may contribute to obesity, a condition related to diabetes and numerous other diseases.

Paradoxically, the fun foods often recommended for inclusion in the diet are notorious sources of refined sugar, fat, saturated fat, and cholesterol. These choices are acceptable because of their high energy value and greater likelihood of acceptance due to their sensory characteristics (Section IV.A.5.b). The reason this paradox exists is that the nutritional and health objectives of PWAs are not the same as for persons without HIV infection.

There are more immediate concerns than the development of chronic diseases that develop slowly over many years. Instead, attention should be focused on the problems of day–to–day eating, especially consuming enough food to maintain a zero or slight positive energy balance and prevent malnutrition, both of which might further compromise immune status in the short run.

TABLE 6
Acceptable Salt Forms of Minerals
for Dietary Supplements

Mineral	Salt form
Calcium	Carbonate
	Dibasic calcium phosphate
	Gluconate
	Lactate
Chromium	Chloride
Copper	(Cupric) sulfate
Iodide	Potassium iodide
Iron	(Ferric) citrate
	(Ferrous) fumarate
	(Ferrous) gluconate
	(Ferrous) sulfate—excellent
	Ascorbic acid chelate
Manganese	Sulfate
Magnesium	Oxide—preferred
Molybdenum	Sodium molybdate
Phosphorus	Dibasic calcium phosphate
Potassium	Supplements not a good source
Selenium	Amino acid chelate—cystine
	Sodium selenite
	Sodium selenate
Zinc	Sulfate

E. DIETARY SUPPLEMENTS

It is a good idea for infected persons to take a high–quality vitamin and mineral supplement on a daily basis. Food supplements vary considerably in quality and potency; cost is not a reliable purchasing guide. It is a good idea to consult a physician for a recommendation. Remember that a supplement is taken to augment the nutrient content of foods contained in the diet, not to replace meals or food groups.

Objective No. 6: *Assure plentiful vitamin and mineral intakes through dietary supplementation.*

Recommendation No 6: *Each day, take a high–quality vitamin and mineral supplement providing at least 100% of the U.S. Recommended Dietary Allowances for essential nutrients.*

There are two criteria for purchasing vitamin and mineral supplements: (1) bioavailability of nutrients and (2) potency. Minerals appear in foods and in supplements in a variety of chemical forms. These forms are treated differently at the gut wall, with some being more readily absorbed than others. For this reason, the bioavailability of minerals is an issue with regard to supplements. Fortunately, vitamins do not appear as salts, and they are treated equally in terms of bioavailability regardless of source—food or supplement.

The salt forms of the various minerals in the supplement determine its quality (Table 6). A high–quality supplement provides minerals with the best chance of getting across your gut wall and into your body. It is important to recognize that the labels of supplements make claims for potency in terms of quantity of mineral present (by weight) relative to the U.S. RDAs (derived from the larger set of RDAs). The claims for potency do not take into account the bioavailability of minerals.

Potency of supplements is a special concern for infected persons, especially those with AIDS and opportunistic infections. There is research with humans to show that high intakes of some nutrients, especially iron, can actually "feed" an infection. Additionally, megadosing of nutrients can lead to toxicity syndromes over time—it is possible to get too much of a good thing. For example, an intake of as little as five times the RDA for vitamin A can result in a chronic toxicity syndrome; therefore, it is important to choose a supplement that provides at least 100% of the U.S. RDA for essential nutrients, but not much more than that level—perhaps 200 or 300% of the U.S. RDA. A doctor should be consulted about the potency of supplements.

REFERENCES

1. American Dietetic Association, Position of the American Dietetic Association: nutrition intervention in the treatment of human immunodeficiency virus infection, *J. Am. Diet. Assoc.*, 89, 839, 1989.
2. **Anon.,** Food guide pyramid replaces the basic 4 circle, *Food Technol.*, 46(7), 64, 1992.
3. **Beisel, W. R.,** Single nutrients and immunity, *Am. J. Clin. Nutr.,* 35, 417, 1982.
4. **Chandra, R. K., Ed.,** *Nutrition and Immunology*, Alan R. Liss, New York, 1988, chap. 1.
5. **Falutz, J., Tsoukas, C., and Gold, P.,** Zinc as a cofactor in human immunodeficiency virus–induced immunosuppression, *J. Am. Med. Assoc.*, 259, 2850, 1988.
6. **Gontzea, I.,** *Nutrition and Anti–Infectious Defense*, S. Karger, New York, 1974.
7. **Hebert, J. R. and Barone, J.,** On the possible relationship between AIDS and nutrition, *Med. Hypotheses*, 27, 51, 1988.
8. Human Nutrition Information Service, *Nutrient Intakes: Individuals in 48 States, Year 1977–78*, U.S. Department of Agriculture, Washington, D.C., 1984.
9. **Jain, V. K. and Chandra, R. K.,** Does nutritional deficiency predispose to acquired immune deficiency syndrome?, *Nutr. Res.*, 4, 537, 1984.
10. **Light, L. and Cronin, F. J.,** Food guidance revisited, *J. Nutr. Educ.*, 13, 57, 1981.
11. **Moseson, M., Zeleniuch–Jacquotte, A., Belsito, D. V., Shore, R. E., Marmor, M., and Pasternack, B.,** The potential role of nutritional factors in the induction of immunologic abnormalities in HIV–positive homosexual men, *J. AIDS*, 2, 235, 1989.

12. **Prasad, C. and Chandra, R. K.,** Nutrition and immunity, in *Gastrointestinal and Nutritional Manifestations of AIDS*, Kotler, D.P., Ed., Raven Press, New York, 1991, 35.
13. **Shoemaker, J. D., Millard, M. C., and Johnson, P. B.,** Zinc in human immunodeficiency virus infection, *J. Am. Med. Assoc.*, 260, 1881, 1988.
14. **Sitrin, M. D. and Rosenberg, I. H.,** Medical and nutritional therapy in malabsorption syndromes, *Drug Ther.*, January, 88, 1979.
15. U.S. Department of Agriculture, *Food for Fitness—A Daily Food Guide,* 3rd rev. ed., Government Printing Office, Washington, D.C., 1977.
16. U.S. Department of Agriculture, *Food Guide for Young Children*, Government Printing Office, Washington, D.C., 1916.
17. U.S. Department of Agriculture, *The Food Guide Pyramid*, Government Printing Office, Washington, D.C., 1992.
18. U.S. Department of Agriculture and U.S. Department of Health and Human Services, *Dietary Guidelines for Americans: Nutrition and Your Health*, Government Printing Office, Washington, D.C., 1990.
19. U.S. Department of Health and Human Services, *The Surgeon General's Report on Nutrition and Health*, Government Printing Office, Washington, D.C., 1988.

Chapter 2

BODY WEIGHT, ILLNESS, AND DEATH

Saroj Bahl

CONTENTS

I. INTRODUCTION

Profound weight loss is a frequent finding in HIV–infected individuals as they progress to acquired immonodeficiency syndrome (AIDS) or AIDS–related complex (ARC). The weight loss seen in these individuals, often severe and progressive, is also accompanied by malnutrition. Wasting and tissue depletion to an extreme degree has been observed in victims of AIDS at autopsy. These characteristic features — wasting, weight loss, and malnutrition — contribute to the clinical dysfunctioning of the immune function, thereby hastening the progression to AIDS and death. The nature of this weight loss, possible causative factors, associated health implications, and nutritional interventions to prevent or retard the tissue depletion comprise the focal points of discussion in this chapter.

A. WEIGHT LOSS

The onset of weight loss, often progressive and severe, may even precede the diagnosis of AIDS. Depletion of body constituents such as fat, protein, intracellular water volume, and potassium has also been noted in AIDS patients. A mean weight loss of 11.81 ± 7.6 kg from the pre–illness usual weight to death was reported in a study by Garcia and associates.[1] Other studies have reported body weight losses ranging from 10 to 33%. The weight loss observed in these patients is accompanied by a chronic depletion of body cell mass. This progressive, relentless wasting has been recognized by the U.S. Centers for Disease Control in Atlanta who have expanded the case definition of AIDS to include the "human immunodeficiency virus (HIV) wasting syndrome". Due to this striking feature of progressive weight loss in AIDS, this disorder has been given the name "slim disease" in Africa (Figures 1 through 3).

B. TIMING OF DEATH

It has been suggested that this progressive malnutrition and weight loss, characteristic of AIDS, may be a factor in the timing of death. Available data indicate that the magnitude of body cell mass depletion rather than its underlying cause determines the timing of death from wasting in AIDS. It has been postulated that a minimal amount of body mass is essential to sustain the vital processes of life, and possibly the weight loss in AIDS patients can exceed that limit. A similar situation exists in other chronic debilitating conditions such as cancer and protein–calorie malnutrition (PCM). Hence, significant conclusions derived from the clinical and nutritional management of these conditions may also apply to AIDS.

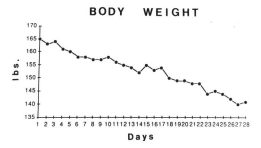

FIGURE 1. Severe and progressive weight loss occurs as HIV infection advances to AIDS or ARC. (From Hickson, Jr., J. F. and Knudson, P., *AIDS Patient Care*, 2(6), 31, 1988. With permission.)

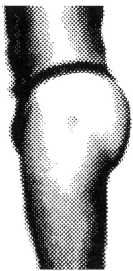

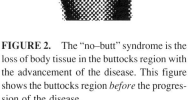

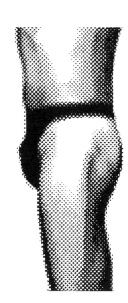

FIGURE 2. The "no–butt" syndrome is the loss of body tissue in the buttocks region with the advancement of the disease. This figure shows the buttocks region *before* the progression of the disease.

FIGURE 3. Loss of body tissue ("no-butt syndrome") in the buttocks region with the advancement of the disease.

A study that was aimed at assessing body weight and nutritional status in AIDS patients reported an average weight loss of 16% from pre–illness weight prior to death. A noteworthy fact revealed by this investigation was that while a large percentage of these patients were malnourished and underweight at the time of admission, the majority did not receive specialized nutritional support during the course of their hospitalization.[2] Based on a review of these studies, it can be concluded that there is a strong possibility that adequate nutritional support of PWA may contribute to maintenance of lean body mass and body weight and thus delay serious complications and death.

II. NATURE AND POSSIBLE CAUSES OF WEIGHT LOSS

Unexplained and unintentional weight loss is usually the first symptom that brings the undiagnosed AIDS patient to the doctor. The development of malignant or infectious complications in patients with AIDS is usually preceded by diarrhea, fever, and weight loss. The presence of Kaposi's sarcoma and weight loss in an HIV–infected individual translates into a poor prognosis for the patient. Cachexia, protein–calorie malnutrition, and severe weight loss seem to coexist in the AIDS patient. The nature and possible factors that may precipitate this state of malnutrition in the AIDS patient need to be understood carefully so that appropriate preventive measures may be undertaken.

A. BODY COMPOSITION

Studies conducted with AIDS patients have indicated that most patients suffering from this disease experience significant depletion of body cell mass, predominantly muscle protein. A greater degree of body cell mass depletion is observed in patients suffering from chronic diarrhea compared to those without diarrhea. Significant depletion of total body potassium and intracellular potassium has been reported; however, the percentage of body weight that is water is increased — a situation that is similar to other states of malnutrition. There is also a relative increase in the volume of extracellular water. Despite the significant depletion in total body potassium, normal or elevated body fat contents are observed in the majority of immunodeficient patients. This state of malnutrition is similar to other conditions of stress such as surgery, trauma, or sepsis. Protein breakdown for energy exceeds catabolism of fat in these situations. The mechanism that promotes excessive protein degradation is poorly understood. To make matters worse, this process may persist despite nutritional therapy.

B. CAUSATIVE FACTORS OF "WASTING" OR WEIGHT LOSS

Weight loss or wasting in AIDS patients has a multifactorial etiology. It may be the end result of a complex interaction of various metabolic, endocrinologic, neuropsychiatric, and gastrointestinal (GI) factors possibly initiated by the HIV infection itself. Several GI opportunistic infections that occur in the AIDS patient, as well as aggressive forms of neoplastic diseases such as lymphoma and Kaposi's sarcoma, are accompanied by severe weight loss.

Oral and esophageal complications that occur as a result of opportunistic infections may impair intake. Like several infections, HIV infection itself may lead to anorexia and reduced intake of food. Anorexia or loss of appetite may result from a number of conditions, which can include neuropsychiatric, endocrinologic, and gastrointestinal. Clinical depression, anxiety, neurosis, and organic brain syndromes associated with HIV infection are included in the category of neuropsychiatric factors. Organic diseases of the brain that are a direct or indirect result of HIV infection can cause loss of appetite. Significant weight loss caused by anorexia and reduced caloric intake also is associated with subacute encephalopathy (HIV–induced subacute encephalitis). In a study conducted with such patients, all of whom had severe anorexia and weight loss, aggressive nutritional support became essential.[3]

Subacute encephalopathy (HIV-induced subacute encephalitis): *Degenerative disease of the brain possibly caused by inflammation resulting from HIV infection.*

Among the endocrinologic factors, adrenal insufficiency has been documented in several studies with AIDS patients. Invasion of the adrenal gland by various infectious agents has also been demonstrated histologically. The exact mechanism underlying these changes is not well understood. Nevertheless, significant weight loss and anorexia have been observed in these patients.

Gastrointestinal infections also contribute to loss of appetite, malabsorption, and resultant weight loss. Several of these infections lead to problems in food intake associated with oral and esophageal complications such as dysphagia, odynophagia, xerostomia, etc. Feeding strategies that may be helpful in alleviating such problems are discussed in Chapter 4. Chronic diarrhea is another common problem encountered in PWA that may cause weight loss. Management of this problem is discussed in Chapter 3.

Still another factor that may contribute to wasting in the AIDS patient is the hypermetabolic state that possibly exists in this disease. Systemic infections such as *Mycobacterium avium-intracellulare,* cytomegalovirus, etc. are associated with hypermetabolism, and most likely the same is true of HIV infection. These conditions and others such as fever and burns are considered classic examples of hypermetabolism and are characterized by increased energy expenditure and protein turnover; however, hypermetabolism can only cause weight loss if energy intake does not match the energy expenditure.

Finally, long–term zidovudine (Retrovir) therapy may be accompanied by weight loss. Symptoms of muscle weakness, tenderness, and atrophy have been reported.

C. WEIGHT LOSS, MALNUTRITION, AND OTHER NUTRITIONAL PARAMETERS

Chronic wasting and weight loss in the AIDS patient imply malnutrition. In addition to loss of body weight, depletion of body cell mass, decreased skinfold thickness and midarm muscle circumference, hypoalbuminemia, and decreased iron-binding capacity have been documented in the AIDS population. Blood levels of prealbumin and retinol-binding protein are also low, and deficiencies of several nutrients such as zinc, selenium, and vitamin B_{12} have been reported. Although the serum levels of these nutrients appear to be subnormal, clinical symptoms of deficiency syndromes have not been documented.

Malnutrition also has been shown to have an adverse influence on immune function (see Chapter 1). It is well recognized that protein–calorie malnutrition has an adverse influence on several aspects of the immune system. Impaired cell–mediated immunity, decreased complement activity, defective phagocytosis, and secretory immunoglobulin production as well as abnormal killer cell function all have been reported in PCM. Hence, this state of malnutrition that is created in the AIDS patient exacerbates the already existing immune deficiency, thereby worsening the course of disease.

III. MECHANISM OF WEIGHT LOSS

Available literature cites several causes of weight loss; yet, the exact mechanism by which the weight loss or wasting occurs is not well understood. It appears that a condition of hypermetabolism, similar to other infectious states, exists. There also appears to be a failure to adapt to the hypocaloric state by adequate metabolic alterations. Malabsorption and diarrhea lead to further deterioration. Malfunctioning of the liver is also present. All of these factors may contribute to the wasting syndrome. However, these are all hypotheses; further research is necessary to elucidate the mechanism underlying the severe weight loss in AIDS patients.

IV. COMPARISON OF WASTING WITH OTHER STATES OF MALNUTRITION

The prevalence of severe weight loss in the AIDS population appears to be almost universal (98%). This contrasts with the approximately 50% incidence of less severe weight loss in some cancer patients. However, in both HIV infection and cancer, the state of wasting can progress to PCM. Development of PCM in the AIDS population is multifactorial and may be caused by inadequate food intake, nutrient malabsorption, and alterations in intermediary metabolism. Since many AIDS–related infections are untreatable, it has been difficult to study the efficacy of nutritional support in malnourished AIDS patients. However, it has been claimed by many investigators, through various case reports, that nutritional support can have a positive influence on quality of life of the AIDS patient.

A. RESEMBLANCE TO CANCER
AND OTHER CHRONIC DISEASES
Loss of lean muscle mass (wasting or cachexia) is a characteristic feature of weight loss in AIDS. A similar situation prevails in other diseases such as cancer and chronic infectious diseases such as tuberculosis. Available evidence suggests that usually deaths in these conditions are caused by progressive

tissue depletion to the extent that life can no longer be sustained. A certain minimum of body mass is essential for the performance of basic bodily functions, such as coughing and clearing pulmonary secretions.

While wasting has been observed in cancer, chronic infectious disease, and AIDS, the mechanisms that cause weight loss appear to be different in these conditions. For example, hypermetabolism has been hypothesized to be one of the possible causes of weight loss in AIDS. However, hypermetabolism is not always observed in cancer patients. Its presence has been demonstrated in conditions of sepsis or burns.

B. RESEMBLANCE TO STARVATION

Some authorities contend that the wasting occurring in the AIDS population is similar to starvation. Studies reported from Northern Ireland about prisoners who imposed starvation on themselves indicated that death occurs when subjects reach approximately 60% of ideal body weight. Similar findings have been reported with AIDS patients. Other data collected during times of food deficits, such as the siege of Leningrad in 1941–1942, reported body weight losses of 37% in the most seriously ill patients. However, studies of semistarvation states have suggested that an average weight loss of 25% is well tolerated.

V. HEALTH IMPLICATIONS OF WEIGHT LOSS

As has been stated earlier, chronic weight loss is associated with malnutrition, which in turn is known to have an adverse influence on the immune system. There is an impairment of cell–mediated immunity. Other adverse effects include lymphopenia, diminished complement concentrations, deficient secretory immunoglobulin production, and defective phagocytosis. These negative effects translate to recurrent episodes of opportunistic illness. AIDS patients may succumb to several infectious agents, including bacterial, parasitic, fungal, and viral agents (see Chapter 1).

A. NUTRIENT DEFICIENCIES

Several nutrient deficiencies have been reported in the AIDS population. In addition, certain deficiencies — particularly those of vitamin A, C, E, and pyridoxine as well as minerals such as magnesium, iron, and some other trace elements — occur in malnourished populations. Depressed serum zinc and thymulin levels have been noted in PWA. Thymulin, a hormone that is involved in immune function, requires zinc for its biological activity. Levels of blood selenium also appear to be lower than normal in AIDS patients. Deficiency of vitamin B_{12} has been demonstrated in HIV–infected individuals as well as AIDS patients. However, the clinical implications of all of these nutrient deficiencies have not been established. Clinical manifestations associated with these deficiencies have not been observed, and the value of supplements also has not been proved.

VI. NUTRITIONAL INTERVENTION STRATEGIES

While the benefits of nutritional support have not been clearly demonstrated in the AIDS population, it is well accepted that nutritional repletion is an important component of the therapeutic regimen in other similar chronic diseases such as cancer. Hence, lessons learned from the nutritional management of cancer and chronic infections such as tuberculosis may find application in the treatment strategy of AIDS patients. Some clinicians have emphasized that drug therapy in the AIDS population is of limited value if it is not combined with adequately designed nutritional support. Effective nutritional therapy promotes a state of homeostasis and enhances the body's response to medical therapy.

A. GOALS OF NUTRITIONAL THERAPY

Nutritional therapy should be aimed at maintaining the general health of the PWA. The primary concerns are maintenance of weight, nitrogen balance, and normal nutritional parameters. These are summarized in Table 1.

There is a great deal of variation between the energy and protein requirements of malnourished ARC/AIDS patients, but both of these requirements are significantly elevated due to metabolic stress. Increased secretion of some hormones (glucagon and catecholamine), elevated proteolysis (breakdown of protein), gluconeogenesis (conversion of proteins into glucose), and ureogenesis (formation of urea) have been reported in metabolically stressed patients. Serum insulin levels are depressed. Due to these metabolic alterations, energy requirements are significantly elevated. Hence, the primary goal of nutritional therapy should be to prevent weight loss.

B. NUTRITIONAL ASSESSMENT

The first step in designing a nutritional care plan for an AIDS patient is to evaluate his/her current nutritional status. The possible causes for unexplained weight loss need to be ascertained. A food diary or calorie count may assist in determining the daily food intake. A patient following an alternative therapy or a fad diet may be suffering from voluntary starvation, or he/she may be experiencing early satiety. The latter may be caused by *Mycobacterium avium–intracellulare* or the presence of neoplastic conditions such as lymphoma and Kaposi's sarcoma.

Weight loss could also occur despite adequate caloric intake. In this case, other possible factors such as the presence of diabetes, drug–induced polymyositis, and infectious agents need to be assessed.

Polymyositis: *Inflammation of several muscles; usually associated with cancer; may be accompanied by pain, edema, tension, insomnia, and sweats.*

TABLE 1
Goals of Nutritional Therapy

Weight management
 Prevent weight loss
 Increase body weight (if underweight)
 Preserve lean body mass

Nitrogen balance
 Maintain positive nitrogen balance
 Prevent protein losses
 Monitor urinary nitrogen losses

Maintenance of normal nutrition parameters
 Maintain total protein, albumin, and transferrin in normal range
 Monitor creatinine/height index
 Monitor total lymphocyte count

Maintenance of normal anthropometric measurements
 Monitor triceps skinfold
 Monitor midarm circumference
 Monitor midarm muscle circumference

Because weight loss in the AIDS patient is often accompanied by PCM, indicators of protein status also should be evaluated. These include serum albumin, transferrin, prealbumin, and retinol–binding protein. In addition, anthropometric parameters such as triceps skinfold thickness, midarm circumference, and midarm muscle circumference should be measured. Nitrogen balance should also be assessed by analysis of nitrogen in a 24–hour urinary urea nitrogen sample.

In general, the guidelines used for nutritional assessment of PWA are similar to those followed for hospitalized and stressed patients. The most frequently encountered problem in such patients is PCM. In these states, the major need is for energy and protein; however, foods that are good sources of protein and energy also provide other essential nutrients. Complete nutritional assessment therefore assists in careful formulation of energy and protein requirements of the AIDS patient. Assessments should be repeated on a weekly basis until nutritional homeostasis (stability) is established.

C. ESTIMATION OF CALORIC AND PROTEIN REQUIREMENTS

Weight maintenance in the general population requires 30 to 35 kcal/kg (usual weight) per day. According to several clinicians, the daily caloric requirement of ARC/AIDS patient is slightly greater, i.e., 35 to 40 kcal/kg (usual weight).[5] For a 70–kg reference man, this would translate to approximately 2500 to 2800 kcal. This level of intake is essential to prevent continued weight loss.

Requirements for protein for ARC/AIDS patients are similar to those of metabolically stressed patients. These individuals require at least 2.0 to 2.5 g/kg (usual weight) of protein per day to maintain a state of positive nitrogen balance. This state contributes to nutritional stability and also prevents loss of body weight.

Individualized dietary regimens based on the recommendations mentioned above should be planned and implemented for ARC/AIDS patients. In addition, regularly conducted blood analyses, nitrogen assessment, and tests of liver function will provide baseline data from which these personalized dietary regimens can be modified. This strategy also assists in the identification of patients who would be good candidates for aggressive nutritional support.

D. FEEDING STRATEGIES

For patients with normal gut function, a high–calorie, high–protein, low–fat, lactose–free oral diet is recommended. In addition, nutritional supplements such as those containing simple carbohydrates, free amino acids, and elemental oral food supplements or resource intact modular food supplements can be used to increase caloric and protein intake. Small, frequent meals may be better tolerated by the anorexic patient. Supplements and snacks may be used to contribute additional calories and protein.

As with the management of other life–threatening illnesses, psychosocial aspects need to be considered. Caregivers need to recognize that just the provision of meals is not sufficient. Because clinical depression is a very common finding in the PWA, emotional support from the caregiver is just as important as the food itself. Personal preferences of food as stated by the patient should be carefully respected. Caregivers also need to communicate the importance of eating to the patient. Other psychosocial factors, such as financial resources, transportation problems, etc., that may impact food–related decisions also need to be addressed.

E. ALTERNATIVE FORMS OF NUTRITIONAL SUPPORT

In certain conditions, where oral feeding is not possible or well tolerated, alternative forms of nutritional support may become essential. Patients with minimal to moderately compromised gut function and moderate to severe diarrhea have been shown to tolerate Compleat Modified Formula (manufactured by Sandoz Nutrition Corp., Minneapolis, MN). This blenderized, meat–based, nasointestinal, enteral diet may not be tolerated well by ARC/AIDS patients with severely impaired gut function. This is possibly due to its lack of low molecular weight free amino acids or polypeptides and high fat content.

In patients who have severe diarrhea, have intermittent or continuous mechanical bowel obstruction, or demonstrate persistent intolerance to oral or nasointestinal enteral diets, parenteral nutrition offers the only hope for survival. Even when given for a short time, parenteral nutrition rests the bowel and helps it to recuperate from any underlying gut infection. Later the patient may be able to tolerate a special oral or nasointestinal enteral diet. However, parenteral nutrition cannot be used for long–term inpatient or outpatient therapy due to its expensive nature.

VII. PREVENTION OF WEIGHT LOSS

"Prevention is better than cure." This statement is very relevant to the HIV– infected individual who still may be asymptomatic. Health professionals should carefully screen all patients with HIV infection, including asymptomatic indi- viduals. Nutritional support should be primarily aimed at maintenance of body weight and preservation of lean body mass. If the HIV– infected individual is underweight, attempts should be made to increase and normalize body weight. Accomplishment of these objectives will require provision of adequate nutri- tion, minimization of malabsorption, and utilization of appropriate feeding strategies. Addressing psychosocial needs of the patient is equally important.

A. NUTRITIONAL STRATEGIES: EARLY INTERVENTION

Early and midstage PWAs may exhibit mild to moderate disinterest in food and all eating behaviors. This may be related to anorexia, which is associated with all chronic infections including HIV infection. Some side effects associ- ated with the medications used to treat the infection also lower appetite. An adequate energy intake will help prevent loss; however, accomplishing this task may be a challenge. Caregivers may need to pay special attention to the patient's food preferences and dislikes as well as presentation of meals.[6]

B. OTHER STRATEGIES

Several other strategies may be helpful in preventing weight loss in the HIV–infected individual. These include adequate drug therapy, with adjust- ments of dosage, timing, etc. as necessary; appropriate and timely treatment of infections; and use of appetite stimulants and other agents that may be helpful in prevention of weight loss. Because research in this area is ongoing, other treatment options may become available in the future.

1. Drug Therapy

Several drugs that are used for HIV–infected individuals may contribute to appetite suppression. Careful adjustment of drug therapy, dosage, and timing of administration may be helpful in reducing anorexia. Recent evidence also indicates that combination therapy (two or three drugs) may be more effective against HIV replication than a single dose; in addition, it may minimize the side effects associated with those drugs (see Chapter 5). Apart from anorexia, many other effects that may reduce food intake have been attributed to drug therapy in HIV–infected persons. These range from mild effects such as nausea and vomiting to serious problems such as hepatic and renal toxicity. Nutritional management of some of these symptoms is discussed in Chapter 5.

2. Treatment of Infections

Recent evidence indicates that some HIV–infected persons with the wasting syndrome may respond to therapy with ganciclovir (dihydroxyphenoxymethyl guanine). This antiviral drug has been known to be effective against cytomegalovirus and other herpes viruses. This finding also indicates that in some patients with HIV infection, untreated infections may be cofactors contributing to catabolic weight loss.

3. Appetite Stimulants

Appetite stimulants such as megestrol acetate, progestins, and estrogens offer some hope for the management of anorexia in HIV–infected individuals. Of these, megestrol acetate shows most promise. This is a steroid used in the treatment of breast cancer that can also improve appetite in AIDS patients suffering from severe anorexia. The effect of progestins and estrogens on appetite has been well known for many years. For example, pregnancy, a state of high progestational activity, is associated with increased appetite and food intake. Further research is necessary to assess the benefits of these appetite stimulants in the AIDS population.

4. Other Agents

Metabolic aberrations associated with AIDS may be reversed with some hormonal agents. For example, oxidation and mobilization of fat appear to be suppressed at the expense of glucose and amino acid oxidation in an infectious illness, and this situation prevails in the AIDS patient. Administration of a growth hormone assists in enhancing fat mobilization and oxidation. It also improves nitrogen balance. Hence, growth hormone therapy may be beneficial in this situation.

Hydrazine sulfate is another agent that has been proposed for use with AIDS patients. This drug can block a catabolic pathway and thereby induce anabolism (formation of new tissue). It has been claimed that hydrazine sulfate therapy in lung cancer patients improves serum albumin, decreases the production of glucose in the liver, and is associated with prolonged survival. However, further research is needed to establish the value of these therapeutic agents in the health management of the AIDS patient.

C. PREVENTION OF OPPORTUNISTIC INFECTIONS

The AIDS patient is a very likely victim for several opportunistic infections. Many of these illnesses are characterized by significant weight loss and fever. Common systemic infections in this category include mycobacterial infections (*Mycobacterium avium–intracellulare* and *M. tuberculosis*), salmonellosis, cryptococcosis, histoplasmosis, and cytomegalovirus. Neoplasms such as Kaposi's sarcoma, lymphoma, and Hodgkin's disease are also characterized by fever and weight loss. Diarrhea, which is a very common symptom of many infections, occurs frequently in the AIDS patient. Hence, adequate therapy of all these conditions is essential for preventing weight loss in the AIDS patient.

D. MANAGEMENT OF NUTRITION–RELATED PROBLEMS

Several nutrition–related problems occur in PWA. These include oral and esophageal pain (see Chapter 4), drug–induced nutritional complications, diarrhea, and malabsorption (see Chapter 3). Nutrition plays a very crucial role in the therapeutic management of these concerns. If not addressed adequately, these problems can cause further deterioration of the patient's health and body weight. However, adequate nutritional management with utilization of appropriate feeding strategies may contribute to stabilization of body weight and prevention of opportunistic illness. A liberal caloric intake that can meet the increased needs of the AIDS patient can only be maintained if all associated nutrition–related concerns are resolved.

VIII. SUMMARY

Weight loss is a frequent finding in ARC or AIDS patients. Several causes, including decreased caloric intake, hypermetabolism, and excessive caloric loss, may contribute to this progressive and relentless loss of body weight. There is a rapid depletion of lean body mass as well. If not corrected, this severe weight loss can lead to early death. Nutrition can perform a crucial role in preventing or decreasing the weight loss and the associated malnutrition that occurs in the AIDS patient. Adequate nutritional assessment and prompt dietary intervention can minimize wasting and replenish lean body mass.

REFERENCES

1. **Garcia, M. E., Collins, C. L., and Mansell, P. W. A.,** The acquired immune deficiency syndrome: nutritional complications and assessment of body weight status, *Nutr. Clin. Pract.*, 2, 108, 1987.
2. **O'Sullivan, P., Linke, R. A., and Dalton, S.,** Evaluation of body weight and nutritional status among AIDS patients, *J. Am. Diet. Assoc.*, 85, 1483, 1985.
3. **Greene, J. B.,** Clinical approach to weight loss in the patient with HIV infection, *Gastroenterol. Clin. N. Am.*, 17(3), 573, 1988.
4. **Kotler, D. P., Tierney, A. R., Wang, J., and Pierson, R. N.,** Magnitude of body–cell–mass depletion and the timing of death from wasting in AIDS, *Am. J. Clin. Nutr.*, 50, 444, 1989.
5. **Hickey, M. S. and Weaver, K. E.,** Nutritional management of patients with ARC or AIDS, *Gastroenterol. Clin. N. Am.*, 17(3), 545, 1988.
6. **Hickson, Jr., J. F. and Knudson, P.,** Optimal eating, Nutrition guidelines for PWAs, *AIDS Patient Care*, 2(6), 28, 1988.
7. **Hellerstein, M. K., Kahn, J., Mudie, H., and Viteri, F.,** Current approach to the treatment of human immunodeficiency virus–associated weight loss: pathophysiologic considerations and emerging management strategies, *Semin. Oncol.*, 17(6) (Suppl. 9), 17, 1990.
8. **Chlebowski, R. T., Grosvenor, M. B., Bernhard, N. H., Morales, L. S., and Bulcavage, L. M.,** Nutritional status, gastrointestinal dysfunction, and survival in patients with AIDS, *Am. J. Gastroenterol.*, 84(10), 1288, 1989.
9. **Hecker, L. M. and Kotler, D. P.,** Malnutrition in patients with AIDS, *Nutr. Rev.*, 48(11), 393, 1990.
10. **Ghiron, L., Dwyer, J., and Stollman, L. B.,** Nutrition support of the HIV–positive, ARC, and AIDS patient, *Clin. Nutr.*, 8(3), 103, 1989.

Chapter 3

CHRONIC DIARRHEA

J. F. Hickson, Jr.

CONTENTS

I. OVERVIEW

A. NUTRITIONAL PERSPECTIVE

Diarrhea is a term meaning "flow of" the intestinal contents, and chronic diarrhea is characterized by occurrences of watery stool day after day. Besides the water loss, the discharge contains all manner of nutrients that did not have an opportunity to be absorbed. Thus, chronic diarrhea can lead to malnutrition. The first priority of treatment, therefore, is to control nutritional losses.

In healthy persons, the usual cause of diarrhea is food poisoning. This condition is better described as a microbial infection of the intestinal canal. It is an infection because living organisms are consumed, usually in contaminated food or drink, and these pathogens go on living in the intestine where they multiply or reproduce. Eventually, the number of microbes present is so large that the organisms can no longer be ignored. The irritated gut wall responds with a dramatic rise in peristaltic activity.

"Peristalsis" is characterized by rhythmic muscular contractions of the gut wall which propel the intestinal contents toward the anus. In food poisoning, the object is to "flush" out the offending microbes. To accomplish this, a dramatic rise in peristalsis results in the very rapid movement (hyperactivity) of intestinal contents out of the body. The result is a watery discharge which may contain recognizable food particles.

The brief episode of diarrhea seen with so–called food poisoning in the healthy person not infected with the human immunodeficiency virus (HIV) usually is not a problem. For example, it is not necessary to take special measures to replenish fluid and electrolytes if there is a reasonable effort made to drink real juices, salted broths or soups, and crackers; together these foods provide water, sodium, and potassium. However, chronic diarrhea can be a serious nutritional problem for persons in the late stages of HIV infection, due to the great losses of water and other nutrients.

B. PSYCHOSOCIAL WELL–BEING

An important aspect of chronic diarrhea is its impact on psychological well–being. Victims of chronic diarrhea often feel "tied to the toilet". This dehumanizing condition occurs when the patient becomes fearful of going anywhere without a toilet nearby because of the possibility of a sudden attack of explosive proportions. Not surprisingly, the second priority of treatment is to give back control over one's body, which provides an increased sense of dignity as well as the freedom to travel outside the home.

One place that a patient might avoid if he/she lacks confidence about bowel activity is the grocery store, yet this is a place that is important to visit in order to buy the food needed to replace losses associated with diarrhea. It stands to reason that a fear of going out to the grocery store can contribute to nutritional decline as much as anorexia or chronic fatigue might reduce the desire to prepare or eat food.

Getting to the grocery store is another problem worth mentioning. Buses, cars, and city sidewalks are not equipped with restrooms. It is easy to imagine how unpleasant it would be to have a sudden, tremendous urge to use the toilet while in the grocery store, while riding in a vehicle, or while walking along the street. What if the patient were to lose control due to the violence of activity in the gut? Of course, it would be very unpleasant. That is the basis for fears of not having a toilet nearby for those who suffer from chronic diarrhea.

II. CLASSIFICATION

Of the general causes of diarrhea, only one results in the production of a high volume of watery stool. The others generally result in diarrhea characterized by small or modest volumes as described below. This difference allows for the classification of diarrhea into two types: low and high volume.

A. LOW–VOLUME DIARRHEA

"Low–volume" diarrhea is characterized by a watery stool, usually less than 1 liter (roughly 1 quart) in volume. Consequently, water and electrolyte losses are going to be modest on a daily basis. This type usually can be treated rapidly and successfully in the typical, healthy adult. No doubt the reader has seen television advertisements for over–the–counter medications (without prescription) that claim to stop diarrhea with a single dose.

Unfortunately, a PWA is not in a condition of typical health. The bowels are diseased with HIV, and it will be necessary to modify expectations for how quickly low–volume diarrhea can be stopped; furthermore, it is important to understand that it will recur again and again. Therefore, treatment is a long–term proposition, a part of a general regimen of health care.

B. HIGH–VOLUME DIARRHEA

"High–volume" diarrhea is characterized by a relatively large, watery stool volume of as much as 10 liters (10.7 quarts) or even more per day. Losses of water and electrolytes are very great on a daily basis due to the tremendous and frequent flushing of the lower gastrointestinal (GI) tract. There is severe malabsorption of all other nutrients indicating major involvement of the small intestine as well.

Generally, high–volume diarrhea does not respond to dietary intervention or withdrawal of food as does the low–volume type. Consequently, this type of diarrhea is considered to be unmanageable or refractory to treatment.

III. CAUSATION

There are at least seven general causes of chronic diarrhea that have been observed in HIV–infected persons. Except in the case of infection with parasites, this serious physical ailment tends to show up after considerable damage to the immune system has occurred. It is thought that the first cause of chronic diarrhea is infection with HIV, which irritates the cells making up the walls of the small and large intestines.

After infection with HIV, the following additional causes of gut infection can be identified: (1) sugar intolerance, (2) a diminished immune system which permits the overgrowth of normal gut flora (microbes) or which does not kill typical levels of foodborne microbes, (3) prolonged use of antibiotics, (4) the effect of chronic diarrhea flushing out the normal, healthy population of microbes in the large intestine, and (5) excessive use of antacids.

Finally, the seventh cause is not caused by the disease, but is only associated with it. In this case, gut tissue is infected with parasites other than the aquired immunodeficiency syndrome (AIDS) virus, foodborne microbes, or microbes that might normally be present in the healthy large intestine.

A. IRRITATION DUE TO HIV INFECTION

Some health care professionals believe that virtually all persons infected with HIV eventually will show signs of gut dysfunction including loss of regular bowel movement activity, abdominal cramping and pain, lactose and fructose intolerance, and chronic diarrhea. Generally speaking, this irritable bowel syndrome due to HIV infection occurs about the time of an AIDS diagnosis after there has been significant damage to the immune system.

To understand how the gut is involved in AIDS, one must realize that it is not just the T lymphocytes of the blood immune system that are involved in the disease. Other body tissues also can become diseased if any of their cells are susceptible to HIV infection.

As AIDS develops over the years, HIV infection progresses throughout the body to include these other body tissues. The portion of the gut that includes the intestines is one which has cells with receptors for the virus making it susceptible to infection; therefore, gut disease and dysfunction might be predicted in virtually all HIV–infected persons who progress to AIDS.

Infected gut cells are irritated by the presence of HIV, and they become hyperactive as a result. With increasing numbers of gut cells becoming infected over time, the level of irritation of all gut cells taken together becomes so great that it interferes with the overall function of the GI tract. When this happens, the symptoms are similar to classic inflammatory bowel diseases seen in persons without HIV infection.

It is not uncommon for physicians to order diagnostic tests of their patients who show symptoms of chronic diarrhea. A typical test is a stool culture to reveal the presence of parasites in the GI tract which may be responsible for the problem. If the findings are negative and no other cause can be found, the problem may be diagnosed as idiopathic diarrhea ("of unknown origin") or AIDS enteropathy (diarrhea due to HIV infection of the GI tract).

B. SUGAR INTOLERANCE

Irritation of the gut wall by HIV infection can lead to its atrophy. Ordinarily the wall of the small intestine is covered with villi: tiny, fingerlike structures that project into the intestinal canal giving the wall a textured, velvetlike appearance (Figure 1). As the wall atrophies, the villi and folds become blunted and flattened; at the extreme they seem to disappear, and the inside surface becomes smooth (Figure 2).

A smooth intestinal wall has a dramatically reduced surface area available for absorption of nutrients including sugars. Another problem is that an atrophied wall does not produce an adequate supply of digestive enzymes for some sugars. Two sugars of special importance are lactose (milk sugar) and fructose (fruit sugar).

These two are only slowly absorbed under the best of circumstances in noninfected persons, and atrophy of the gut wall only serves to make their

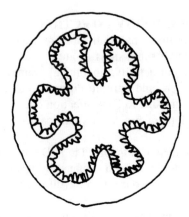

FIGURE 1.   Cross section of the small intestine for a healthy individual illustrating extensive wall folds and fingerlike villi projecting into the canal to maximize surface area for nutrient absorption.

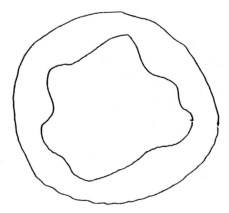

FIGURE 2.   Cross section of the small intestine illustrating the effect of inflammatory bowel disease on the wall; as drawn here, the wall folds and villi that should project into the canal are atrophied, becoming blunted and flattened and leaving a smooth surface of reduced absorptive area.

digestion and absorption even slower. The problem is that unabsorbed sugars remaining in the gut canal too long will cause "osmotic" diarrhea by attracting water from inside the body. Once enough water has accumulated inside the canal, the flushing syndrome of diarrhea begins.

C. IMPAIRED IMMUNE SYSTEM

Chronic diarrhea can result from diminished capacity of the immune system consequent to AIDS. In the healthy individual, the intestinal tract is protected from infection by a variety of immune factors including immunoglobulins

(IgA) that are secreted directly into the canal. In the small intestine, these factors control the activity of microorganisms consumed with foods, preventing them from becoming a problem.

Gut wall secretion of immune factors is also important for the microbial populations of the large intestine. Microbes in the large intestine are prevented from moving up into the small intestine by this system. Additionally, overgrowth of microbes in the large intestine is resisted. When microbes are not checked, they may produce irritating by–products leading to diarrhea.

D. PROLONGED USE OF ANTIBIOTICS

The prolonged use of antibiotic drugs can lead to chronic diarrhea. Such treatment can lead to ulceration of the gut wall, and irritable bowel syndrome can follow. Again, irritable bowel syndrome can cause diarrhea due to hyperactivity of the gut — foods and beverages move through the intestinal canal too quickly to be absorbed (Section III).

A second problem with chronic antibiotic use is that it kills off the populations of "favorable" microorganisms (flora) that normally are present in the large intestine of a healthy individual. Favorable microbes are those that do not produce by–products which irritate the gut wall and cause diarrhea.

"Good" microbes normally predominate over the "bad" ones in the large intestine, preventing the bad ones from gaining a foothold. Unfavorable microorganisms can cause changes in bowel activity including gas production (flatulence) and diarrhea. When the population of favorable microbes in the large intestine is reduced due to the chronic use of antibiotics, the unfavorable ones have an opportunity to establish themselves and wreak havoc.

The possibility of unhealthy changes in gut flora with antibiotic administration is but one of several reasons why physicians are reluctant to prescribe freely antibiotics to persons infected with HIV. It should be expected that access to these drugs will be more limited than for persons who are not infected.

E. FLUSHING EFFECT OF CHRONIC DIARRHEA

Just like the chronic use of antibiotics, chronic flushing (diarrhea) of the large intestine can wipe out the normal presence of favorable microorganisms (Section III.D). This loss can lead to unhealthy changes in bowel activity because unfavorable microbes are not suppressed, and they may establish colonies.

Unabsorbed or undigested nutrients coming from the small intestine into the large intestine serve as food for these unfavorable microorganisms. Irritating by–products of metabolism are produced, which can lead to diarrhea and gas.

F. CHRONIC USE OF ANTACIDS

Antacids are commonly used to relieve "stomach distress" or "acid indigestion". Some persons get into the habit of using these drugs; they might be used in connection with therapy involving other AIDS drugs that might irritate or damage the stomach walls, making them highly sensitive to acid. Antacids provide relief by "absorbing" acid.

This is contrary to the normal function of the stomach during its processing of food. An acidic stomach environment serves important functions, one of which is to protect against the typical, low–level microbial contamination of foods. Acid kills disease–causing, pathogenic and nonpathogenic micro-organisms including all three fungi — bacteria, molds, and yeasts — as well as viruses.

Chronic and/or heavy use of antacids raises the pH (decreases the acidity level) of the stomach, making it an ineffective barrier to microbes. This failure can result in infections of the stomach. Furthermore, microbes may pass to the intestines where they can cause infections.

Importantly, pathogens as well as nonpathogens both may be infective organisms leading to diarrhea. This problem is compounded by impaired immune function in HIV–infected persons (Section III.C).

G. PARASITIC INFECTION

Chronic diarrhea due to parasitic infection has been linked with AIDS because it was a common affliction in the male homosexual (gay) community; furthermore, AIDS first came to the attention of health professionals as a gay disease. Hence, chronic diarrhea of parasitic origin was associated with AIDS, but this does not mean that parasites cause AIDS.

Several intestinal parasites causing diarrhea have been identified. Those that have been observed in immunocompromised persons include *Shigella*, *Cryptosporidium*, *Isospora belli*, *Enterocytozoon* or *Giardia lamblia*. Contact with infected fecal matter has been the usual mode of transmission from person to person; *Shigella* is particularly infectious. These microorganisms are not the "garden variety" normally found in the healthy, lower gut. Additionally, they are not representative of foodborne pathogens causing food poisoning such as *Salmonella*, *Campylobacter*, *Staphylococcus*, *Vibrio*, and *Clostridium*.

The manner in which these parasites infect and irritate the GI wall leads to the large volume of water losses. The membrane permeability of cells lining the intestinal canal is altered. Consequently, water readily moves out of the body into the canal leading to a flushing phenomenon, and this type of diarrhea is usually termed "secretory".

Unlike other causes of diarrhea, this one has to be managed by a physician. Ordinarily, the physician will make a culture of the person's stool in order to confirm parasitic infection and to identify the organism. Once the causative parasite has been identified, then the doctor will select a drug to kill it.

It should be recognized that parasitic infection may be cured. However, underlying problems that were masked may now be exposed including HIV infection of gut tissue leading to chronic diarrhea (Section III.A).

IV. NUTRITIONAL CONSEQUENCES

A. LOW–VOLUME DIARRHEA
1. Irritation Centered in the Small Intestine
The area of the bowel affected determines the specific nature of the nutritional consequences for low–volume diarrhea. Energy–yielding nutrients (protein, fat, and carbohydrate) as well as vitamins and minerals (other than electrolytes) are absorbed in the small intestine, the portion of the GI tract between the stomach and large intestine. When irritated due to HIV infection, the absorption of these nutrients is reduced.

a. Protein
It is important to recognize the role of protein in providing energy because it is commonly thought to be exclusively used in tissue construction as a structural component. Furthermore, malabsorption of protein contributes to the atrophy of skeletal muscle tissue associated with AIDS.

When the quality and quantity of amino acids (protein) being absorbed across the gut wall are insufficient to meet daily needs, then the body will raid its own protein "reserves", mainly skeletal muscle tissue. Raiding a reserve has negative consequences because the functional capacity of the body is reduced, and a reserve cannot be repleted simply by refeeding. Two important outcomes from raiding protein reserves include atrophy and weakness of skeletal muscle tissue.

b. Carbohydrates
Malabsorption of carbohydrates causes two major problems. First, carbohydrates provide roughly 43% of calories for typical Americans each day. Hence, weight loss rapidly results when it is not absorbed because of the large energy deficit. Unfortunately, the weight being lost is not restricted to adipose (fat) tissue. Inadequate energy intake will increase the use of protein as a source of fuel. This protein can come from the diet or body tissues; when it comes from body tissues, then atrophy of skeletal muscle results.

Yet another problem with carbohydrate malabsorption is that the unabsorbed nutrient will move down the gut where it can be fermented by the microbes normally inhabiting the large intestine. This can produce not only flatulence (gas), but also a variety of breakdown products that may further aggravate the GI tract and result in even more diarrhea.

c. Fat
Malabsorption of fat also leads to a large energy deficit because typical Americans derive about 41% of calories from this nutrient. Again, weight loss is not restricted to adipose tissue. Inadequate total energy intake can increase the use of protein for fuel including that from internal sources leading to atrophy of skeletal muscle tissue.

The movement of undigested fat into the lower gut can result in steatorrhea or "fatty stools". The stool is cream–colored or very light brown.

d. Vitamins

The loss of vitamins in the stool due to malabsorption at the small intestine is of little consequence in the short run (days). The reason is that the body generally maintains "stores" of vitamins when the typical American diet is routinely consumed. Stores are supplies that can be depleted and repleted to meet the needs of the body without resulting in negative consequences. This is the reason that brief bouts of diarrhea in healthy persons generally do not impact vitamin status.

Both fat– and water–soluble vitamins are stored. For fat–soluble vitamins A, D, E, and K, body stores may amount to 3– to 12–month supplies. In contrast to popular wisdom, the stores of water–soluble vitamins can be substantial when the typical American diet is consumed. For example, the vitamin C store can last for 2 to 4 months, and the vitamin B_2 store can last for 2 to 6 months.

When diarrhea continues over the long run, vitamins are not absorbed in sufficient quantity to meet the body's daily requirements and maintain the various stores. When this occurs, deficiency diseases can develop. It is a good idea for your physician to be on the lookout for symptoms of these diseases because they are no longer a common (i.e., widespread) nutritional/health problem in the United States, and they may not be recognized for what they are.

e. Minerals

Minerals such as iron, zinc, calcium, and magnesium, but excluding electrolytes, are found in reserves like protein instead of stores like vitamins. Again, reserves can be utilized as a source of nutrients to meet demands, but negative consequences may result in terms of the body's capacity to function. Furthermore, the repletion of reserves can be difficult or impossible to achieve. For example, the bone can be considered to be a reserve for calcium that has been built up over many, many years. Depletion of calcium from the bone results in "soft" bones or osteomalacia, a condition that may be irreversible.

The mineral reserves are quite substantial relative to daily needs. The body can sustain long periods — weeks, months, and even years — with insufficient intakes of certain minerals. For this reason, malabsorption of minerals is not an immediate concern for short–run diarrhea as would be the loss of two electrolytes, potassium and sodium. On the other hand, preventive measures are appropriate for chronic diarrhea with continuing losses.

2. Irritation Centered in the Large Intestine

Ordinarily, water and electrolytes (sodium and potassium) are mostly absorbed in the large intestine, the part of the GI tract that follows the small intestine and terminates at the anus. When the large intestine is irritated due to HIV infection, this absorption process is disrupted and significant losses can occur.

a. Water Deficiency

While the daily loss of water for low–volume diarrhea is considered to be moderate at about 1 l (a little less than a quart), it can become very important if it is not fully replaced each day. When not replaced, losses are said to "accumulate". Water is unique among nutrients in that its accumulated losses produce negative consequences very fast, in a matter of just 1 or 2 days.

Water deficiency or dehydration is the result of accumulated losses of water. When dehydrated, the body cannot properly control its temperature, blood pressure, or heart rate. These effects can be seen with a loss of as little as 2 to 3% of body weight as water.

Body temperature rises in the dehydrated state because there is insufficient water available to permit adequate heat loss through sweating, the most important mechanism for cooling the body. Sweating, particularly through evaporation at the skin surface, carries away from the body enormous amounts of heat into the air. When heat builds up inside the body because it cannot be sweated away, then the safe operating temperature range is exceeded and systems begin to fail.

Decreased blood volume results in a drop in blood pressure. This impairs the body's ability to deliver oxygen and nutrients throughout the body. At the same time, it becomes more difficult to rid the body of waste products. It is the kidney's job to clean the blood and form urine in the process. This organ is dependent on blood pressure created by the pumping action of the heart to force blood though it for filtration. When pressure falls, blood flow is reduced and waste products build up in the blood to toxic levels.

Physical performance is impaired for several reasons. Decreased capacity to sweat means that the heat produced at the working muscles cannot be removed; as heat accumulates, the muscles lose the capacity to function. Heart rate is another limiting factor. Due to the decrease in blood volume, the heart rate rises to compensate (tachycardia); however, when an individual exercises, the heart rate has to increase in order to service the working skeletal muscle tissues, so the potential for it to rise further with exercise is reduced. The result is a decreased ability to engage in any type of exercise, possibly even light activity around the house.

b. Electrolyte Losses

Electrolytes are electrically charged particles. All are derived from mineral elements. Of the 16 different electrolytes, 10 are positively (+) charged and 6 are negatively (–) charged. Two of the most abundant and important electrolytes are sodium and potassium.

These two electrolytes have several roles in the body. Both govern the distribution of water in the various body fluid compartments or spaces of the body. Specifically, sodium maintains the volume of the blood while potassium holds water inside the cells of tissues including the skeletal muscle. Additionally, both electrolytes are involved in the transmission of electrical impulses within nerves. Like water, electrolyte losses can accumulate rapidly, in only a few days depending on the severity of diarrhea.

In the early stages of sodium depletion, fluid shifts occur among compartments. The problem is that water tends to move out of the blood into the skeletal muscle cells. As with dehydration, the decreased blood volume results in a fall in pressure. The heart attempts to make up for this problem by pumping faster. Typical symptoms include headache, lightheadedness, mental dullness, loss of appetite, muscular weakness, and muscle cramps, among others.

Potassium deficiency also occurs rapidly with chronic diarrhea. A major concern is a reduction in the sensitivity of heart and skeletal muscle to nervous stimulation. At the heart, this results in abnormal beating patterns. Even worse, the characteristic rhythm of the heartbeat may be lost, resulting in death of heart tissue and possibly a life–threatening crisis for the individual.

B. HIGH–VOLUME DIARRHEA
The nutritional consequences of chronic, high–volume diarrhea are essentially the same as for the low–volume type except that deficiency syndromes develop much more rapidly and are more difficult to control. Dehydration and loss of electrolytes are the overriding concerns.

V. NUTRITIONAL TREATMENT

A. LOW–VOLUME DIARRHEA
Even when low–volume diarrhea cannot be stopped entirely, a careful strategy of oral feedings can be successful in getting energy, water, and other nutrients inside the body, and crisis situations can be avoided. You will want to develop a strategy involving more than one approach to the problem of diarrhea. Again, diarrhea in the person with HIV can be a multifactorial problem of a continuing nature. By combining several approaches, you will "cover all the bases". Several approaches are described in this section.

1. Dietary Strategy
A person's diet encompasses both the specific foods consumed and the nutrients contained in those foods. In treating diarrhea, it is necessary to consider each of these factors separately. Getting the required nutrients into the body is the goal of a sound diet strategy that includes a variety of foods; however, some food vehicles are better tolerated than others due to the way in which nutrients are present. Additionally, foods are subject to contamination with microbes, and food sanitation is more important for the PWA than for the noninfected person (Chapter 6).

2. Nutritional Intake
The need for a nutritionally adequate diet is of general importance in AIDS to prevent malnutrition. The same considerations are applicable to combat the

effects of chronic diarrhea with the exception that water and electrolyte replacement is of special concern. General aspects of nutritional treatment have been presented in Chapter 1, Section IV; additional discussion regarding energy and protein nutrition is given in Chapter 2. Water and electrolyte replacement, specific to chronic diarrhea, is discussed below.

3. Water and Electrolytes

The loss of water can easily be made up by drinking fluids. Foods can also contain significant amounts of water even though they appear to be solid. It is a good idea to drink plenty of real fruit juices and eat fresh fruits not only because they are good sources of water, but also because they are excellent sources of potassium.

The front label on juice products should be read carefully. Products called "fruit punch" or "fruit drinks" are not the nutritional equivalents of real fruit juices. These formulated beverages can be poor sources of potassium. Despite their names, they may contain little or no real fruit juice. Read the label for nutritional contents.

Orange juice can serve as a meaningful reference standard against which to compare other products regarding potassium value. It contains about a whopping 500 mg (0.5 g) of potassium per cup.

While real juices are generally good sources of potassium, they are poor sources of sodium, having only a few milligrams per cup. Sodium losses can be replaced very easily by salting food during preparation and at the table. Regular table salt can be used liberally unless otherwise instructed by the doctor. This is an example of one of the nutritional paradoxes that exist for HIV–infected individuals. The third edition of the "Dietary Guidelines for Americans"[11] recommends "avoiding too much sodium". This guideline is based on a link by association, but not by causation, between sodium intake and the development of hypertension in humans.

B. HIGH–VOLUME DIARRHEA

Large amounts of water and electrolytes are lost each day with high–volume diarrhea. These losses rapidly accumulate to become life threatening. Modern oral rehydration therapy (ORT) or oral rehydration solution (ORS) is designed to replace both water and electrolytes. Research and development of ORS occurred after World War II and continued through the 1960s.

ORS contains three basic components: water, sodium, and potassium. It was discovered that the passive uptake of sodium across the intestinal wall is linked to the active uptake of glucose and/or amino acids; therefore, ORS with glucose and/or amino acids is more effective in delivering sodium. Potassium is very readily absorbed from the gut.

A standard composition of ORS has been established by the World Health Organization (WHO)/UNICEF. This standard provides optimal concentrations and safe solutions for use in practical, unsupervised settings.

Dehydration should not be treated with water alone. The untreated electrolyte imbalances will result in convulsions and water intoxication leading to death. Similarly, salt replacement without water has severe consequences. This indicates the importance of solutions that have been properly designed; in particular, soft drinks are not a good choice since they are often devoid of sodium. The WHO/UNICEF ORS is considered optimal and can be obtained through physicians.

It is not considered safe to make rehydration solutions in the home. Precise measuring equipment is needed to prevent even small errors in the added quantities of sodium and potassium. Additionally, the person preparing the rehydration solution must be trained in order to make measurements correctly. Folk recipes do exist, but their effectiveness has been called into question.

VI. SUGAR INTOLERANCE

Sugar intolerance in persons who were previously tolerant is secondary to HIV–induced irritation of the GI tract. These symptoms can be expected to occur in many HIV–infected persons, particularly those with AIDS for which there has been significant progression of the disease at the gut (Section III.A). The traditional rule in the management of sugar intolerance is to avoid consumption of the foods and/or beverages that contain the sugars causing diarrhea. Another way to manage sugar intolerance, as in milk, is to reduce portion sizes at mealtime.

A. LACTOSE

Milk sugar, lactose, is comprised of two subunits, glucose and galactose. When the gut wall is atrophied and/or irritated, its production of lactase, the digestive enzyme for milk sugar, is not adequate. This leads to accumulation of lactose molecules in the small intestine. In turn, the lactose molecules draw water from the body into the gut canal; once enough water has accumulated, then diarrhea results.

In the past, the traditional dietetics approach was to eliminate all foods containing lactose. In effect, milk products were omitted from the diet. This proved to be unacceptable, though, because milk is an excellent source of calcium and riboflavin as well as a good source of protein among other nutrients.

It has been learned that many persons who show lactose intolerance can still consume milk products, but portion sizes have to be reduced. For example, one cup of fluid milk might not be tolerated, but one half cup may do just fine.

A folk wisdom that has not been proved states that yogurt and other fermented products are lactose–free and therefore can be consumed as desired. In fact, fermented milk products can contain significant amounts of lactose leading to diarrhea.

The modern way to handle lactose intolerance is to take advantage of developments in food technology that have yielded preparations of concentrated lactase enzyme. Milk is treated by dropping liquid concentrate into the carton, shaking well, and then waiting overnight before drinking the milk. The extent of lactose breakdown depends on how many drops of solution were added. The taste of milk changes noticably because the presence of free glucose gives a sweeter taste than the larger molecules of lactose. Yet, the taste remains mild and pleasant.

Solid dairy products are treated in a different fashion. After the first bite of the product, one or more pills of lactase enzyme concentrate are eaten. Then the rest of the dairy product is eaten. The number of pills needed varies with an individual's capacity to digest lactose. In this case, there is no effect of treatment on the taste of the food. The lactase enzyme is widely available in drugstores as an over–the–counter preparation.

B. FRUCTOSE

Fructose causes diarrhea in the same manner as lactose. This fruit sugar is not assisted in its absorption across the gut wall into the body. Consequently, it moves in only slowly. Damage to the gut wall due to HIV further slows absorption. This allows fructose to accumulate in the gut canal. From there it draws water into the gut leading to diarrhea.

You may first report fructose intolerance after making a connection between diarrhea and the consumption of orange juice. This juice, which contains fructose, is a familiar component of American breakfasts; hence, it is more likely to be consumed than other fruits.

The problem is not unique to orange juice; any fruit with a significant amount of fructose can cause diarrhea. In general, to avoid fructose–induced diarrhea, avoid the consumption of fruits in large servings. Through a trial and error method, the appropriate portion sizes for favorite fruits will be determined.

VII. TREATMENT WITH DIETARY FIBER

A. INTRODUCTION

No doubt you have seen television commercials for dietary fiber, a dietary aide that is supposed to soften the stool and improve the "regularity" of bowel movements. There are many kinds of dietary fiber, but in general they can all be grouped as either soluble or insoluble. The soluble type of dietary fiber is important for the treatment of diarrhea.

Soluble dietary fiber attracts water and binds with it tightly to form a jellylike substance in the gut canal. The water available for binding with the dietary fiber may come from a meal or from intestinal secretions. You can think of soluble dietary fiber as acting like a sponge. Since it is considered undesirable to take water from the body, food manufacturers may recommend that water or other beverage be consumed with their dietary fiber product.

When the dietary fiber molecules swell, they add "bulk" to the feces. In other words, the size of the fecal matter is greater, but more importantly the water content has increased. The feces are now softer and easier for the body to move and eliminate (Section VIII.E). Hence, the constipation is relieved and regularity can be achieved.

The HIV–infected person can also make use of soluble dietary fiber, but in a different way. In this case, the objective is exactly the opposite from a healthy person seeking regularity in bowel function or softness of stool. The HIV-infected person would consume soluble dietary fiber with a minimum of liquid. As it moves through the GI tract, it soaks up water, preventing its accumulation in the large intestine, which would lead to diarrhea. Additionally, the dietary fiber and the water it has attracted may combine with fecal material to create more fecal material. In these two ways, soluble dietary fiber may stop diarrhea temporarily.

While dietary fiber is not a drug, it is still important to respect this food supplement. If taken in excess, it can have such a drying effect that constipation will result or the bowels might even become clogged or impacted. In general, dosage suggestions on the product label should be followed. Experiment carefully in small steps, and keep a log of dosages and dates. Try to correlate this information with bowel activity. The objective is to determine the smallest effective dose.

B. PSYLLIUM

One potentially effective source of soluble dietary fiber is psyllium. This plant product can be purchased at the drugstore in various forms. One popular form is lightly sweetened wafers or cookies wrapped in foil to preserve freshness (Metamucil Fiber Wafers, Procter & Gamble; Cincinnati, OH). For best results, the product label directions specify that 1 to 2 cups of hot or cold beverage should be consumed with each dose of two wafers. Keep in mind that these directions were not written for HIV–infected or AIDS patients; they were intended for persons who want to soften their stool rather than to make it firm.

Patients might want to try eating the wafers without liquid. The psyllium will soak up the water in the lower gut instead of the water that was recommended for drinking. The result is a drying effect at the large intestine that could stop diarrhea until the next bowel movement when the "plug" is lost. Then the process will have to be repeated.

The product label directions indicate that up to three doses may be taken each day, but this recommendation assumes that a beverage is consumed at the same time. Caution is advised to prevent overdrying of the gut canal. Consumption of the product without beverage is not how it was intended to be used. Instead, experiment with the product for different applications.

Unlike drug therapy (Section VIII), the use of soluble dietary fiber probably has little or no effect on reducing nutrient malabsorption since the gut tissue remains hyperactive. Cumulative nutrient losses are still a source of concern.

C. BRAN

Wheat bran is an example of a source of insoluble dietary fiber. It does not combine with water to make a jellylike substance in the gut canal. Instead, the "physical presence" of bran against the gut wall stimulates peristalsis, which reduces fecal transit time. Physical presence relates to the fact that bran consumed in sufficient quantity can take up significant space in the canal and make sufficient contact with the wall to elicit nervous impulses. In turn, the information conveyed by nervous transmission to the brain and back to the gut increases the coordinated muscular activity of peristalsis. This is contrary to the patient's need where the gut is already too active.

D. PECTIN

Pectin, used to make fruit jelly, is another well–known source of dietary fiber. Pectin is not a good choice to aid in the control of diarrhea because it is fermented (i.e., consumed as a nutrient source) by the microbes normally present in the large intestine. Furthermore, pectin supplements may actually lead to diarrhea through the formation of products that irritate the lower gut wall.

E. LOW–RESIDUE DIET

Ironically, while some health care professionals are now experimenting with psyllium to control diarrhea, "low–residue" diets have traditionally been recommended. The low–residue diet is one that produces little fecal bulk (volume of feces). The justification for it was that the physical presence of feces and the bulk–producing agents in the gut canal stimulated bowel activity. Hence, traditional dietetics emphasized "partial" bowel rest through the recommendation of a diet consisting of refined foods.

Accordingly, animal products including beef, poultry, fish, milk, cheese, and butter, which do not contain any dietary fiber, were acceptable for eating. By contrast, plant products (i.e., fruits and vegetables), which do contain dietary fiber, were not acceptable, with the exception of refined wheat flour used to make "white" bread. Prior to the introduction of antidiarrheal drugs (Section VIII), the low–residue diet may have been attractive in its capacity to reduce the volume and/or severity of diarrhea, but it could not stop the problem altogether.

VIII. DRUG THERAPY

A. INTRODUCTION

Generally speaking, the modern antidiarrheal drugs are not intended to be used in the treatment of chronic diarrhea. These medications are for use in the rare occasions of simple diarrhea in otherwise healthy individuals. In the noninfected person, drug treatment according to label directions is generally effective. By contrast, long–term drug therapy may be required for irritable bowel syndrome when the root problem, HIV infection, cannot be cured. Long–term treatment is really experimental in nature. For this reason, the patient and doctor should work together when antidiarrheal drugs are used as therapy.

Of the medications available, some require a physician's prescription while others can be purchased in the pharmacy as "over–the–counter" preparations. In either case, it is important to remember that drugs can have powerful and unanticipated effects. A doctor should be consulted before beginning drug therapy to select the drug and work out a course of therapy together.

B. CONTRAINDICATIONS

The use of any antidiarrheal drug is inappropriate when the gut canal is infected with foodborne microbes or parasites transmitted through sexual practices, or when the normal flora from the large intestine are overgrown and/or have moved up into the small intestine. When the gut is infected in these ways, it is desirable that the flushing action of diarrhea continue in order to wash out toxic by–products.

C. SELECTION OF A DRUG

Normal gut tissue displays gentle peristaltic contractions, which slowly propel food material from the small intestine into the large intestine and then toward the anus. By contrast, HIV–infected gut tissue is irritated and hyperactive as a result. Drugs that affect gastrointestinal motility are popular and widely used to reduce the activity level of irritated tissue in order to stop diarrhea.

These drugs act through the bloodstream on smooth muscle tissue of the GI tract, putting it to "sleep" temporarily. In this calm state, water has the opportunity to be absorbed from the gut canal, particularly from the large intestine. This stops diarrhea, and relatively normal looking feces may even develop; however, when the drug wears off, diarrhea will resume if not checked again by continued therapy.

Opiates are a class of drug in this category that have a long history of effectiveness as demonstrated by common observation. Of these, the synthetic opiate, loperamide (McNeil Consumer Products Co., Fort Washington, PA; also manufactured and/or licensed by Janssen Pharmaceutica Inc., Piscataway, NJ), has been very well received. The following attributes of loperamide should be noted: it is (1) widely available (does not require a doctor's prescription), (2) affordable, (3) rapid acting, (4) well tolerated, (5) nonaddictive, and (6) administered in "pill" form. These are ideal characteristics for a drug to be used in long–term therapy.

Importantly, loperamide has been suggested in the relief of chronic diarrhea due to inflammatory bowel disease. This is exactly the medical problem that HIV infection presents.

Other drugs besides loperamide, notably diphenoxylate and codeine, are available; however, undesirable side effects have been reported with their use.

D. DOSAGE

The dosage is something to be worked out with the physician. Generally speaking, a dose level that effectively controls diarrhea and improves quality of life is desired. Common experience suggests that effective doses vary tremendously. As a general rule, it is most desirable to take the minimum effective dose to establish consistent relief from day to day. If the patient ends up on a rollercoaster ride, going from diarrhea to constipation (Section VIII.E) and back, then the therapy has not been correctly applied. Each individual must work with the doctor to find the correct regimen; one person's routine will not work for everyone (Tables 1 and 2).

E. CONSTIPATION

The duration of the drug effect depends on the dose administered. Some report that very small doses of loperamide work for one or two days, while higher doses can stop bowel movements altogether for several days at a time.

Despite any perceived benefit of great freedom from the toilet on days of inactivity, it is a good idea to avoid high doses because they can result in the formation of "dry" and "hard" fecal matter in the large intestine. This feces is termed dry because its water content is low, and hard because its texture is overly firm.

Ordinarily, the gentle peristaltic contractions of the large intestine are sufficient to move feces along the canal providing that they possess the right amount of "wetness" and "softness". These properties are necessary in order for the feces to move down the intestinal canal consequent to the pushing and mashing actions of the smooth muscles of the gut wall.

Under the influence of an excess dose of loperamide, the level of peristaltic activity is too low for too long, particularly at the very end of the large intestine before the rectum. The feces formed in this location under the effect of the drug have too much opportunity to surrender water content to the body and then become dry and hard as a result.

When the drug wears off, peristaltic activity resumes. Yet, attempts to move the dry, hard feces out of the large intestine into the rectum for holding before evacuation are not met with success.

Compounding the problem, soft and/or watery fecal material has accumulated far behind the plug of dry, hard feces. The physical presence of this fecal

TABLE 1
Diary Entries of a Case Report Showing an Early Experiment with Loperamide to Gain Control Over Diarrhea in a Person with AIDS

Date	Description of bowel movements (BMs)	Loperamide administration[a]
10/31/91	6 BMs, all diarrhea	10 mg in 3 doses
11/01/91	None	2 mg
11/03/91	None	
11/04/91	None	
11/05/91	None	
11/06/91	None	
11/07/91	1 BM, good volume, well-formed, dark brown	

[a] Minimum dose was 2 mg.

TABLE 2
Diary Entries of a Case Report Showing the Practiced Use of Loperamide to Maintain Regularity of Bowel Activity Without Diarrhea in a Person with AIDS (GI Tract Completely Evacuated on the First Day — 10/10)

Date	Description of bowel movements (BMs)	Loperamide administration[a]
10/10/92	4 BMs, firm and dark (1), soft (1), very soft (2), last 3 light brown	None
10/11/92	None	4 mg in 2 doses
10/12/92	1 BM, very soft, light brown	2 mg
10/13/92	None	None
10/14/92	None	None
10/15/92	1 BM, firm, large, well-formed, dark brown	None
10/16/92	None	None
10/17/92	1 BM, moderately firm, large, poorly formed, medium brown	None
10/18/92	None	None

[a] Minimum dose was 2 mg.

TABLE 3
Microorganisms Present in
Selected Dietary Supplements

Bifidobacterium adolescentis
B. longum
Lactobacillus acidophilus
L. casei subspecies *rhamnosus*

material in the canal stimulates the gut walls to continue contracting. With each contraction there is dull pain in the lower abdominal area, around and below the naval. An individual, infected or not, who has this experience is "constipated".

IX. TREATMENT WITH FAVORABLE MICROORGANISMS

It is a folk remedy to "recolonize" or reestablish the gut microflora after a course of diarrhea that may have flushed or washed part of the microflora away. Accordingly, normal bowel activity may be restored in healthy persons by recolonizing the gut with favorable microbes.

According to the folk remedy, persons recovering from bouts of diarrhea should drink lots of buttermilk or eat lots of cultured milk products. These dairy products contain live microbes such as lactobacilli that are considered to have favorable activity in the gut. They are the so–called "good" microbes of the gut.

To recolonize the large intestine, the diet is supplemented with many billions of favorable microbes. It is easy to do this because there are a variety of milk products with live cultures on the market (for example, buttermilk and yogurt). In addition, concentrated supplements in pill or capsule form are available, particularly in health food stores (Table 3).

X. FOOD SANITATION

Food sanitation is of great importance with regard to diarrhea. Many bouts of diarrhea among healthy persons are due to consumption of food that is highly contaminated with microorganisms. As discussed previously, ingested live microbes produce irritating by–products that cause movement of water into the GI tract and hyperactivity of the gut muscles. Together, these conditions result in diarrhea.

In healthy persons, the immune system and the flushing response are rapidly successful in ridding the body of the offending microbes, but immunocompromised persons may not be as fortunate since it takes fewer microbes to cause illness in them. Pathogens and nonpathogens both can cause illness; in the healthy individual, though, the nonpathogen might not be a problem. Furthermore, the compromised integrity of the GI tract lining may provide access for microbes into the bloodstream, resulting in an infection throughout the entire body.

Care must be taken to observe proper sanitation in making food purchase decisions, storage, preparation, cooking, and serving of food to prevent infections transferred by food. This topic is discussed in more detail in the context of defensive eating in Chapter 6.

XI. CHRONIC USE OF ANTACIDS

Chronic use constitutes abuse. Although antacids can be purchased without a prescription, they are drugs and they are not harmless. If you need antacids on a regular basis, then it is time to consult you doctor to determine whether there is an appropriate alternative.

REFERENCES

1. American Dietetic Association, Position of the American Dietetic Association: nutrition intervention in the treatment of human immunodeficiency virus infection, *J. Am. Diet. Assoc.*, 89, 839, 1989.
2. Food and Nutrition Board, *Recommended Dietary Allowances*, 10th ed., National Academy, Washington, D.C., 1989.
3. **Gracey, M., Ed.,** *Diarrhea*, CRC Press, Boca Raton, FL, 1991.
4. **Keusch, G. T. and Farthing, M. J. G.,** Nutritional aspects of AIDS, *Annu. Rev. Nutr.,* 10, 475, 1990.
5. **Kotler, D. P.,** Diarrhea in AIDS: diagnosis and management, *Resident Staff Physician,* 33(10), 30, 1987.
6. **Kotler, D. P.,** *Gastrointestinal and Nutritional Manifestations of the Acquired Immunodeficiency Syndrome*, Raven Press, New York, 1991.
7. **Kotler, D. P., Scholes, J. V., and Tierney, A. R.,** Intestinal plasma cell alterations in acquired immunodeficiency syndrome, *Dig. Dis. Sci.,* 32(2), 129, 1987.
8. **Riecken, E. O., Zeitz, M., and Ullrich, R.,** Non–opportunistic causes of diarrhoea in HIV infection, *Bailliere's Clin. Gastroenterol.* 4(2), 385, 1990.
9. **Sachs, M. K. and Dickinson, G. M.,** Intestinal infections in patients with AIDS, *Postgrad. Med.,* 85(4), 209, 1989.
10. Task Force on Nutrition Support in AIDS, Guidelines for nutrition support in AIDS, *Nutrition* 5(1), 39, 1989.
11. *Dietary Guidelines for Americans: Nutrition and Your Health,* U.S. Department of Agriculture and U.S. Department of Health and Human Services, Washington, D.C., 1990.

Chapter 4

ORAL AND ESOPHAGEAL COMPLICATIONS: NUTRITIONAL MANAGEMENT

Saroj Bahl

CONTENTS

I. INTRODUCTION

Nutritional management of the acquired immunodeficiency syndrome (AIDS) patient represents a challenge to all health care professionals. First identified in 1981, AIDS is known to be caused by the human immunodeficiency virus (HIV). AIDS is the last or final stage of HIV infection or disease and is characterized by several symptoms caused by "opportunistic" infections.

Opportunistic infections: *Caused by germs that take advantage (or opportunity) of the weakened immune system and cause diseases that a healthy body could resist.*

Some of these symptoms involve the oral (mouth) and esophageal (related to esophagus or gullet) tissues. Hence, feeding of the AIDS patient becomes very difficult. Yet, adequate intake of nutrients is essential for maintenance of the health of AIDS patients. This chapter will discuss the various types of infections and other causes of oral and esophageal complications and their nutritional management.

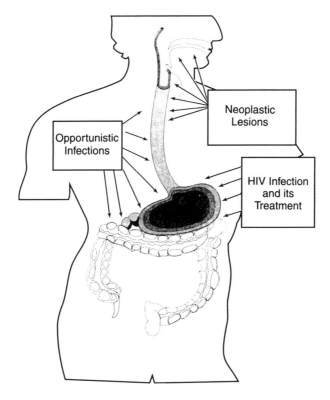

FIGURE 1. Gastrointestinal tract of the AIDS patient.

A. AIDS AND THE GASTROINTESTINAL TRACT

Studies indicate that the gastrointestinal (GI) tract is a major target organ for AIDS–related disease. Involvement of the oral cavity (mouth area), esophagus (gullet), stomach, small and large intestines, and the liver has been reported. Gastrointestinal complaints were indicated by 85% of the patients in a study by Crocker.[1] Increased sensitivity of the gastrointestinal tract is possibly due to the effects of the primary systemic disease: HIV infection, which affects the entire body, and its associated treatment, as well as invasion by opportunistic pathogens (germs that cause disease) and neoplasms (any new and abnormal growth) (Figure 1).

B. COMMON GASTROINTESTINAL COMPLAINTS
   ## IN THE AIDS PATIENT

Common gastrointestinal complaints reported by the AIDS patient are listed in Table 1. Such complaints lead to wasting of protein and reduced dietary intake. Intake of food is further compromised by the presence of pain in the mouth and esophageal area as a result of Kaposi's sarcoma (KS), *Candida* and cytomegalovirus, or herpes virus infections. Oral and esophageal pain is

TABLE 1
Common Gastrointestinal Complaints
in the AIDS Patient

Anorexia (poor appetite)
Nausea/vomiting
Abdominal pain
Steatorrhea (fat in the stool)
Lactose intolerance (inability to tolerate milk sugar)
Changes in taste sensation
Difficulty in chewing and swallowing

associated with chewing problems, dysphagia (difficulty in swallowing), or odynophagia (painful eating).

C. INCIDENCE OF GASTROINTESTINAL — ORAL AND ESOPHAGEAL — COMPLICATIONS IN THE AIDS PATIENT

A chart review of 80 patients with AIDS indicated that 32 (40%) experienced oral and esophageal complications such as candidiasis, dysphagia, and odynophagia. In another study, oral candidiasis was reported in 94% of patients with AIDS. These oral complications are accompanied by several feeding problems, some of which are listed in Table 2. In addition, the therapeutic interventions utilized in the AIDS patient may be accompanied by nausea, vomiting, and decreased appetite. Such complications may also result from infection, fever, emotional stress, and drug–related effects. However, with an individualized approach of nuritional intervention and dietary modification, adequate intake of food can be maintained.

D. TYPES OF ORAL AND ESOPHAGEAL COMPLICATIONS IN THE AIDS PATIENT: CAUSES, SYMPTOMS, AND TREATMENT

The various types of oral and esophageal complications that occur in the AIDS patient are summarized in Table 3. Commonly noted symptoms of these conditions and nutritional management strategies are also given. Several opportunistic infections have been known to affect the gastrointestinal tract in the AIDS patient. These include fungal, viral, bacterial, and protozoan infections. In addition, neoplasms (abnormal growth of tissue), the most common being Kaposi's sarcoma (KS), lead to oral and esophageal complications. Other oral lesions may result from gingivitis (inflammation of the gums) and periodontal disease, salivary gland enlargement, idiopathic thrombocytopenic purpura, and oral ulceration.

Idiopathic thrombocytopenic purpura: *Purplish, brownish discoloration of the skin due to decrease in blood platelets; cause unknown.*

TABLE 2
Feeding Problems Related to Oral
and Esophageal Complications
in the AIDS Patient

Esophagitis (inflammation of the esophagus)
Xerostomia (dryness of the mouth)
Limited production of saliva
Dysphagia (difficulty in swallowing)
Odynophagia (painful eating)
Dysgeusia (changes in taste)
Aspiration
Obstruction

II. OPPORTUNISTIC INFECTIONS

A. FUNGAL: *CANDIDA* SPECIES

One of the frequent causes of oral and esophageal lesions in the AIDS patient is a local invasive infection caused by *Candida* species. In a study conducted by Barr and Torosian[3] with patients suffering from AIDS, 94% of the subjects had oral candidiasis. This condition produces pain and reduces the flow of saliva.

Candida albicans is a common commensal fungus that is a normal inhabitant of the human alimentary tract. Less common species, including *C. tropicalis, C. parapsilosis,* and *C. krusei*, occur infrequently in the normal alimentary tract, but they predominate in the immunocompromised patients who have received broad–spectrum antibiotics. Proliferation of *Candida* within the alimentary tract is encouraged by the diminished concentration of competing bacteria from the normal flora which results from the use of broad–spectrum antibiotics. The oral cavity and esophagus are the most common gastrointestinal sites that are affected by the AIDS–related *Candida* infection. Esophageal candidiasis and most other cases of candidiasis appear to develop from the normal flora of the alimentary tract.

1. Oral Candidiasis

Oral candidiasis may occur in several forms, all of which may occur in association with HIV infection. Primarily, there are three types of oral candidiasis: angular cheilitis, atrophic candidiasis, and pseudomembranous candidiasis.

Angular cheilitis: *Condition characterized by ulceration (broken tissue), cracking, fissuring, and reddening of the skin around the corner of the mouth.*

TABLE 3
Oral And Esophageal Complications in the AIDS Patient:
Causes, Symptoms, and Nutritional Management

Causes	Common symptoms	Nutrition management
OPPORTUNISTIC INFECTIONS		
Fungal		
Candida albicans	Dysphagia	Avoid spicy foods
	Dysgeusia	Use mechanically softened
	(defective taste)	foods served at room
	Ulceration	temperature
	Bleeding	
	Decreased salivation	Use candy or peppermint to
	Nausea	improve taste
	Esophagitis	Avoid any other foods that
		cause discomfort
Viral		
Cytomegalovirus	Dysphagia	Avoid spicy
	Odynophagia	foods/irritants
	(painful eating)	Use mechanically softened
		or pureed foods served at
		room temperature
Herpes simplex virus	Painful ulceration	Avoid any foods that
	Dysphagia	cause discomfort
	Esophagitis	Use mechanically softened,
		pureed, or blenderized
		high–protein foods
Human papilloma virus	Oral papillomas (warts)	Maintenance of oral hygiene
	Warts over other	is important
	parts of body	Avoid acidic, salty, spicy,
		coarse and crunchy, or
		rough foods
Varicella virus	Unilateral pain	
(herpes zoster)	Ulceration	A liquid or soft diet
		is well tolerated
Epstein–Barr virus	Oral lesions (on the lateral	Maintenance of oral hygiene
(hairy leukoplakia)	margins of the tongue,	is important
	buccal mucosa, etc.)	Avoid acidic, salty, spicy,
		coarse and crunchy, or
		rough foods
		A liquid or soft diet is well
		tolerated
Protozoan		
Cryptosporidium	Dysphagia	Avoid spicy foods/irritants

TABLE 3 (continued)
Oral And Esophageal Complications in the AIDS Patient:
Causes, Symptoms, and Nutritional Management

Causes	Common symptoms	Nutrition management
Bacterial *Mycobacterium avium–intra–cellulare*	Oral lesions—palatal and gingival	Use mechanically softened foods served at room temperature Eat foods that are served at room temperature
NEOPLASMS		
Kaposi's sarcoma	Sore gums, ulcers, obstruction	Frequent mouth rinses may be helpful
Non–Hodgkins lymphoma	Dysphagia	Increase consumption of high–protein foods Use mechanically softened foods served at room temperature
OTHER LESIONS		
Gingivitis and periodontal	Severe pain, loosening of teeth; ulcers at interdental papillae	Avoid spicy and acidic foods Eat a high–protein, high-calorie liquid diet until tissue health is restored
Oral ulceration (Hormonal factors, food allergy)	Ulcers that become large and necrotic; very painful	Progress to soft diet
Enlargement of salivary gland	Xerostomia (dry mouth)	Use artificial saliva and sugarless lemon drops Consume a liquid diet or high-moisture foods (tea with lemon, gravies, sauces, Popsicles®, sherbet, etc.)

Atrophic candidiasis: *Atrophic form of candidiasis occurring as a red lesion that may be found on the hard and soft palate (roof of the mouth) and at the back of the tongue.*

> **Pseudomembranous candidiasis:** *Condition also termed as oral thrush in everyday language; characterized by the presence of creamy, curdlike plaques or patches that occur on the oral mucosa (lining tissue of the mouth); removing these patches often reveals a bleeding surface.*

It has been shown that oral candidiasis in association with HIV infection may be a common forerunner of AIDS. The condition has also been used as a marker for esophageal candidiasis, thereby providing sufficient documentation for the diagnosis of AIDS according to Centers for Disease Control guidelines.[1] Other disorders that may also lead to esophageal candidiasis include diabetes mellitus, hypoparathyroidism, and adrenal insufficiency.

2. ESOPHAGEAL CANDIDIASIS: SYMPTOMS

Involvement of the esophagus results in severe dysphagia (painful swallowing), which in turn causes diminished dietary intake. Symptoms of esophageal candidiasis include bleeding and ulceration (inflamed, broken tissue). In addition, odynophagia (painful eating) and retrosternal pain (pain behind the anterior thoracic wall) have been noted. However, the most common gastrointestinal symptom associated with oral and esophageal candidiasis is dysphagia.

Presence of these various lesions in oral and esophageal candidiasis leads to difficulty in chewing and swallowing. Also, the condition may persist for several weeks if left untreated. In severe cases of candidiasis, eating and drinking may become a very painful and practically impossible task. Hence, accurate diagnosis of candidiasis followed by effective treatment is crucial.

3. Treatment of Oral and Esophageal Candidiasis

A number of therapeutic strategies have proven effective in the clinical management of oral and esophageal candidiasis. Topical antifungal medications and systemic drugs (taken internally that affect the entire body) have been found to be effective. Factors such as compliance (or the patient's compliance) and other underlying medical problems may determine the choice of therapy. Treatment may include antifungal drugs such as clotrimazole (Mycelex®), ketoconazole (Nizoral®), amphotericin B (Mysteclin F®), and acyclovir (Zovirax®). (Refer to Chapter 5.) Oral medications include clotrimazole and nystatin (Mycolog II®) tablets, which are available in different dosages, flavors, and textures that can be adjusted as needed.

B. VIRAL INFECTIONS

Among the opportunistic infections that may invade the HIV–infected patient are several other viral infections. These are cytomegalovirus (CMV), herpes simplex virus, human papillomavirus, and varicella virus. General symptoms of these viral infections are fairly similar and range from painful lesions to dysphagia and odynophagia.

1. Cytomegalovirus

Cytomegalovirus attacks the gastrointestinal tract of the AIDS patient thereby leading to direct mucosal damage (damage to the intestinal wall) and further infection of the sensitive tissue. Characteristic features of this infection include diarrhea (with or without blood), fever, weight loss, abdominal pain, and distention. Oral and esophageal pain, chewing difficulties, odynophagia, and dysphagia are also present.

Cytomegalovirus is treated with intravenous administration of ganciclovir (DHPG–9®, manufactured by Syntex Laboratories, Inc.). Life–long therapy may be required because aggravated recurrence of the infection is likely if the treatment is discontinued. This treatment is also accompanied by loss of appetite and nausea, which may make feeding even more difficult.

2. *Herpes Simplex Virus*

Painful ulcers are a characteristic feature of this viral infection. The lesions caused by the infection may occur on the gums and the palate (roof of the mouth). A sudden appearance of small blisters on these surfaces is followed by their rupture resulting in painful ulceration. Lesions or ulcers can also occur on the tongue, making it difficult to distinguish from other diseases with similar symptoms. Hence, confirmed diagnosis is only possible with cytological smears or cultures of early lesions. Oral acyclovir administered several times a day is an effective form of treatment.

Cytological smear: *A specimen of cells spread across a glass slide; examined for the origin, structure, function, and pathology of the cells.*

---

3. Human Papillomavirus

This viral infection is characterized by the occurrence of warts, several different types (oral papillomas) that may appear on many different parts of the body. These warts may have a flat surface or show as multiple fingerlike projections covered with horny cells. Such multiple growths may be scattered throughout the oral cavity. Recurrence of the warts following surgical removal has been noted.

4. Varicella Virus

Another member of the herpes group is the varicella virus which causes herpes zoster. This infection produces characeristic skin lesions and oral ulcerations that are usually quite painful. In the early phase, small blisters may occur in the mouth; these rupture and heal without any significant problem. However, when these blisters occur on the external surfaces of the skin, they become "crusted" and are usually painful. Complaint of a tooth pain, without any obvious dental cause may be one of the early symptoms.

5. Epstein–Barr Virus

This virus causes a white lesion that occurs predominantly on the lateral margins of the tongue (sides of the tongue). This lesion represents a unique feature of HIV–infected patients and is a significant clinical indicator or early warning sign of HIV infection.

The lesions of oral hairy leukoplakia, which were first observed in male homosexuals in 1981, have been noted in all other risk groups for AIDS, including children. In this infection, white "creamy"–looking patches occur on the tongue and on the buccal (cheek) and labial (lips) mucosa (mucous membranes lining these organs). Hairlike projections may appear from the thickened surface of the skin. While the condition may interfere with dietary intake, it is usually asymptomatic. Complete resolution of this infection can be achieved with the experimental drug desciclovir, an analogue of acyclovir (Zovirax®) which is used for the treatment of herpes zoster.

C. PROTOZOAL INFECTIONS

Some protozoal infections associated with AIDS–related gastrointestinal disease include *Cryptosporidium, Isospora belli,* and *Giardia lamblia.* These are not foodborne infections, and most of the microbes invade both the small and large bowel. Among these, *Cryptosporidium* needs to be discussed because it may sometimes cause dysphagia that interferes with normal feeding.

1. Cryptosporidium

This protozoan usually leads to a severe, debilitating nonbloody, high–volume type of diarrhea (refer to Chapter 3). Other symptoms are weight loss, malabsorption, and abdominal cramping. Mortality associated with this condition is high, and no treatment has proved to be consistently effective. Esophageal inflammation and dysphagia have also been observed in patients suffering from this infection. Therapy of this infection may be primarily aimed at maintenance of fluid and electrolyte balance and parenteral nutritional support.

Esophageal inflammation: *Refers to localized, protective response initiated by trauma or breakdown of tissue; in this case, affecting the esophagus or gullet.*

D. BACTERIAL INFECTIONS

Several foodborne bacteria, such as *Salmonella, Shigella, Campylobacter,* and *Mycobacterium avium-intracellulare* (MAI), may infect the gastrointestinal tract in the AIDS patient. Most of these microbes cause low–volume, osmotic diarrhea and associated disease. However, MAI has been known to cause clinically significant oral lesions. This microbe rarely causes disease in healthy persons; however, it causes fever, weight loss, malaise (vague feeling of bodily discomfort), and diarrhea in the AIDS patient. In addition, it may cause ulcerated mucosal lesions on the palate and gingiva (gums). Although these oral lesions rarely occur as a result of this infection, a few cases have been reported by Volpe et al.[6]

III. NEOPLASMS

AIDS–related neoplasms include Kaposi's sarcoma and non–Hodgkin's lymphoma. Both of these neoplasms may influence the functioning of the gastrointestinal tract. Oral manifestations have also been observed in both types of neoplasms.

Neoplasm: *New, abnormal growth of tissue; progressive and uncontrolled.*

A. KAPOSI'S SARCOMA

Historically, this neoplasm was first reported as occurring in elderly, middle-aged Jewish or Mediterranean men in the 19th century. Recently, it has been observed in East Africa. In these groups, the lesions had a slow growth and responded readily to therapy; however, the lesions of Kaposi's sarcoma (KS) are aggravated by HIV infection and are sometimes quite resistant to therapy.

Early lesions of Kaposi's sarcoma occur in the mouth area. The hard palate is the site affected most commonly. The early lesions may be flat or raised and can range in size from smaller than a millimeter to large nodules. They can be red, blue, or purple in color. When the lesions occur on the gingival surface (gums), the condition may resemble periodontal disease. These KS lesions may become inflamed and quite painful, thereby compromising dietary intake. Occurrence of the lesions in the esophagus leads to esophagitis (inflammation of esophagus) and dysphagia. Treatment of KS is done with chemotherapeutic agents such as vinblastine (vinkaleukoblastine sulfate), radiation therapy, and laser therapy. No matter what therapeutic strategy is employed, however, the lesions will recur several months after treatment.

B. NON–HODGKIN'S LYMPHOMA

This may appear as a painless lesion that can occur anywhere in the oral cavity. Swelling and ulceration may follow, possibly from trauma. Both intestinal and esophageal lymphoma have been reported. Dysphagia may occur when esophageal lymphoma is present.

Lymphoma: *Refers to any neoplastic (abnormal growth) disorder of the lymphoid tissue.*

IV. OTHER LESIONS

A. PERIODONTAL DISEASE AND GINGIVITIS

In general, periodontal disease is believed to be associated with bacterial infections that result in the destruction of supporting structures of the teeth. However, the presence of certain chronic diseases increases the risk of periodontal disease: diabetes, leukemia, hyperparathyroidism, or hypoparathyroidism.

Individuals infected with HIV exhibit a tendency to develop severe inflammation of the gums and progressive destruction of supporting structures of the teeth. The condition progresses very rapidly in the HIV–infected individuals, thereby leading to degeneration of alveolar bone (bony sockets to which teeth are attached), periodontal ligament, and associated tissues. Also, severe pain, more so than in non–HIV–infected patients, has been observed. Offensive bad breath accompanies periodontal disease in HIV–infected patients. The underlying cause of these lesions and bacterial flora that lead to periodontal disease in HIV–infected patients is not well understood at this time.

B. SALIVARY GLAND DYSFUNCTION

While the cause is unknown, swelling of the salivary glands, usually the parotid glands, has been reported in children and adults with HIV infection. The primary complaint associated with enlargement of the salivary glands is xerostomia (dry mouth).

C. ORAL ULCERS

Several individuals (without HIV infection) report the occurrence of small red ulcers in the mouth area. These are called "recurrent aphthous ulcers" (RAU). Although the precise cause underlying their appearance is unknown, possibly hormonal factors, food allergies, stress, and viral factors are involved. These recurrent ulcers occur with increasing frequency in individuals with HIV infection. Sometimes these lesions are extremely large, painful, and necrotic (broken, dead cells). To make matters worse, these ulcers may persist for several weeks in HIV patients.

V. DIETARY MANAGEMENT OF ORAL AND ESOPHAGEAL COMPLICATIONS IN THE AIDS PATIENT

A. GENERAL GUIDELINES

1. Objectives of Dietary Management

Objectives of dietary management in a patient suffering from oral and esophageal complications related to AIDS are twofold:

- To maintain an adequate intake of calories, protein, vitamins, and minerals
- To provide foods that can be ingested with minimal pain and discomfort

2. Modifications in Food Consistency and Texture

To achieve the first objective, modifications in food consistency and texture may be beneficial. Liquid or semiliquid food can help stimulate the flow of saliva. If poor swallowing coordination is a problem, thickening of the liquids may be helpful. For individuals who suffer from aspiration, semisolid consistency of foods may be ideal. It is generally recommended that the PWA should select foods or food combinations that have a uniform consistency and that form a cohesive bolus in the mouth and pharynx. Selection of foods that have high energy and high protein is necessary to meet these objectives.

3. Types of Foods and Feeding Strategies

Ideally, soft, nonirritating foods served at room temperature should be used. Hot, acidic, salty, or spicy foods as well as hard foods such as pretzels, hard bread, and potato chips should be avoided. Foods that stick to the palate (e.g., white bread, peanut butter) and slippery foods (e.g., jello, macaroni) should be avoided. Drinking of liquids should be accomplished with straws. Appropriate therapeutic regimens aimed at alleviating mouth pain and mucous membrane trauma should be used. These can include the administration of systemic pain medications prior to meals, eating Popsicles®, and use of a xylocaine rinse before mealtimes. Optimal oral intake is also facilitated with the maintenance of good dental hygiene. In cases where dysgeusia (alteration of taste) is present, adjustments in texture and temperature will improve appetite, salivation, and acceptance of food. Production of saliva is enhanced with liquids and carbohydrate foods such as gum and candy. Control of nausea and vomiting can be accomplished by eating small, frequent meals; using easily digested foods, and avoiding fatty, greasy, and spicy foods.

Common symptoms of most opportunistic infections that affect the AIDS patient can be summarized as dysphagia and odynophagia, esophagitis, xerostomia, dysgeusia, stomatitis (painful ulceration), and gingivitis. Specific dietary strategies aimed at addressing some of these specific symptoms will now be discussed.

B. MANAGEMENT OF SPECIFIC SYMPTOMS

1. Dysphagia and Odynophagia

The term "dysphagia" refers to any problem in chewing or swallowing foods, beverages, or medications. The most serious health risk associated with dysphagia is aspiration. The irritation caused by food particles that fall into the trachea and the lungs encourages aspiration pneumonia and other pulmonary infections. Hence, the patient should be instructed on swallowing techniques that prevent food from being aspirated.

Signs of dysphagia include drooling, collection of food in the mouth, feeling of "lumps" in the throat; choking or coughing associated with swallowing efforts; and a wet, "gargly–sounding voice" or hoarse breathing. When pain is present — generally associated with infections, neoplasms, and obstructions — the condition is called "odynophagia".

Nutritional management of the dysphagia patient necessitates the following recommendations:

- Modifications in food texture and consistency
- Adjustments in food temperature
- Selection of adequate foods
- Adjustments in patient's position

Mechanically softened foods, pureed or blenderized, should be used. Because thicker liquids are more easily managed than thin liquids, alter the consistency of thin liquids by adding gelatin, pureed fruits, yogurt, or commercial thickening agent. Foods that form a cohesive bolus should be used (e.g., pureed chicken, souffles, tuna salad, puddings, etc.). The swallowing reflex is stimulated by certain textures, e.g., toast rather than bread. Foods close to room temperature are better tolerated and accepted. Provision of high–kilocalorie, high–protein supplements is helpful in improving the nutritional status of the patient. Adequate positioning of the patient is important. The patient should be seated upright, in a comfortable position with the head slightly tilted forward. Also, encourage the patient to keep sitting for at least half an hour after eating. When the patient does lie down, the head of the bed should be elevated 6 inches at all times. The principles underlying managements of dysphagia (and odynophagia) are summarized in Table 4.

Some individuals may have a problem with excessive mucus production. Suggestions for controlling formation of mucus include:

- Use adequate amounts of fluids.
- Withhold milk, particularly if lactose intolerance is observed. As an alternative, yogurt can be given to the patient.
- Use of some juices (e.g., pineapple, grapefruit, and cranberry) may be helpful. These juices help decrease the production of mucus.

TABLE 4
Management of Dysphagia/Odynophagia
Nutritional and Other Considerations

Nutritional considerations

Select a variety of foods, particularly high–kilocalorie and high–protein supplements

Avoid spicy foods, especially when pain is present

Use mechanically softened, pureed, or blenderized foods that make a "cohesive bolus"

Consistency of thin liquids can be altered by adding gelatin, yogurt, or
commerical thickening agents

Eat foods that are served at room temperature

Other considerations

Patient should sit upright when eating

Do not recline for at least 30 minutes or longer after eating

Keep bed elevated 6 in. at all times

Control mucus formation

Use juices such as grapefruit

Take liberal amount of fluids

Use mucus–thinning agents, e.g., papain and warm–air vaporizer

Withhold milk (use yogurt instead)

- Mucus–thinning agents, such as papain (an enzyme found in papayas), can be beneficial. These can be applied locally (on a glycerin swab) before eating or taken as tablets.
- A warm–air vaporizer can be used. This helps to thin mucus.

2. Esophagitis

Esophagitis (inflammation of the esophagus) can occur in the lower or upper part of the esophagus. Factors that contribute to development of esophagitis include infectious organisms, chemical and physical agents, and trauma. Nutritional deficiencies, particularly those of iron and B–complex vitamins, may lead to inflammation of the upper esophagus (Plummer–Vinson syndrome). A common symptom is heartburn, a burning epigastric substernal pain.

Heartburn: *Severe, burning sensation occurring in the upper middle region of the abdomen, beneath the sternum.*

TABLE 5
Management of Esophagitis:
Nutritional and Other Considerations

Nutritional considerations

Foods to be avoided

High–fat foods (decrease fat to less than 45 grams/day)

Alcohol, peppermint, coffee, tea, and chocolate (these foods decrease LES pressure)

Irritants, e.g., citrus, juices, spicy foods, carbonated beverages

Any other foods that cause discomfort

Foods to be increased

High–protein foods

Nutrient supplements as needed (iron and vitamin B complex)

Other considerations

Do not recline for 2 hours after eating

Do not wear tight-fitting clothing

Eat small, frequent meals

Avoid constipation

Do not take fluids with meals

Esophagitis is caused by chronic esophageal reflux (backing up of stomach contents into the esophagus) which in turn is related to reduced lower esophageal sphincter (LES) pressure. Many factors influence LES pressure, one of which is hormonal control. For example, the frequent occurrence of heartburn during pregnancy may be explained by decreased LES pressure, which is related to elevated levels of progesterone.

Lower esophageal sphincter: *A sphincter (a ringlike band of muscle fibers that constricts a passage or closes a natural orifice) situated at the junction of the esophagus and stomach (lower end of esophagus).*

Nutritional care of esophagitis is aimed at decreasing irritation to the esophagus, increasing LES pressure, decreasing the volume and frequency of reflex, and last, but not least, increasing the clearance of digestive materials from the esophagus. Other considerations such as posture of the patient, frequency of meals, and avoidance of constipation are also important. General principles underlying the management of esophagitis are summarized in Table 5.

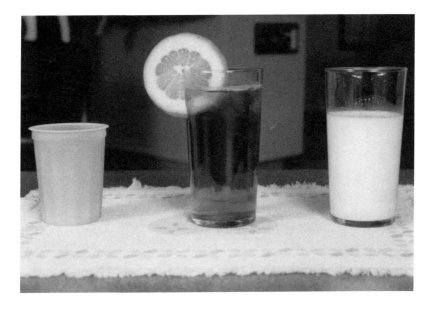

FIGURE 2. Recommended use of glycerine-and-lemon mouthwash and generous intake of fluids for patients suffering from xerostomia.

3. Xerostomia

This condition, which refers to "dryness of the mouth", can result from abnormalities in salivary function or factors that affect fluid or electrolyte balance. Adequate nutritional management of xerostomia is crucial because studies have linked this condition with malnutrition. Xerostomia has a notable impact on the ability to lubricate, masticate, tolerate, and swallow certain foods. Perception of taste is significantly affected.

Nutritional care of patients suffering from xerostomia should be aimed primarily at maintaining moisture in the mouth. This can be achieved by several measures such as the use of a glycerine–and–lemon mouthwash and generous intake of fluids or hard, sugarless candies. Production of saliva can be increased by the use of artificial saliva, glucose polymers, and saliva stimulants such as sugarless lemon drops and gum. Maintenance of oral hygiene and frequent saline rinses are also helpful. Dry foods, bread products, meats, crackers, bananas, and excessively hot foods may not be well tolerated. Also, alcohol is poorly tolerated and should be avoided. Foods with high moisture content should be encouraged: gravies, sauces, casseroles, sherbet, citric acid-containing foods, melons, vegetables with sauces, and meats such as chicken and fish. Fruit juices, fruitades, carbonated beverages, Popsicles®, and tea with lemon are also recommended (Figures 2 and 3).

4. Dysgeusia

The term "dysgeusia" refers to a distortion in taste perception (alterations in sense of taste). This symptom can occur in the HIV–infected patient as a

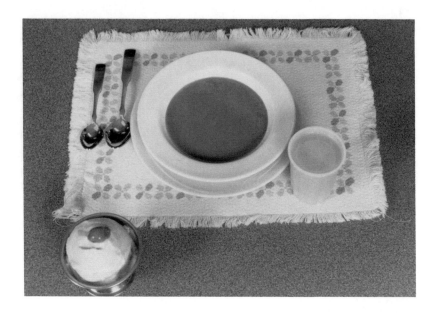

FIGURE 3.   Recommended diet of high moisture content for patients suffering from xerostomia.

result of some opportunistic infections and as a side effect of some medications (rifabutin, pentamidine, etc.). Certain nutrient deficiencies such as those of zinc, B vitamins, and vitamin A have also been associated with taste alterations.

Maintenance of good oral hygiene, including rinsing of the mouth before eating, is fundamental in the management of dysgeusia. Improvement of taste perception can be achieved with the use of sour candy or peppermint. An individualized approach to feeding the patient is desirable. In general, certain foods such as greasy or fried foods, red meats, chocolate, coffee, and tea are poorly tolerated. Acid foods such as fruit-flavored supplements are beneficial because they stimulate taste. Foods should be served at room temperature.

5. Stomatitis, Sore Mouth, and Painful Ulcers

These conditions, which can make eating very difficult, can occur in HIV–infected patients as a consequence of several fungal, viral, or bacterial infections. In addition, neoplasms and gum disease also can lead to soreness in the mouth area.

Management of ulceration or soreness in the mouth area involves several strategies. Medications such as analgesics or pain killers can reduce or alleviate the discomfort associated with eating. Frequent saline rinses and maintenance of oral hygiene are also helpful. As far as dietary recommendations are concerned, a liquid or soft diet is generally well tolerated. Foods such as broth–based soups, fruitades, carbonated beverages, and melons are well accepted. Extremes of temperature in serving food should be avoided. Also, acidic, salty, spicy, coarse and crunchy, or rough foods are not well tolerated. A straw should be used whenever possible.

6. Gingivitis and Periodontal Disease

These dental problems can also occur in non–HIV–infected individuals; however, HIV infection further complicates the situation and aggravates these symptoms. Gingivitis can occur in a severe form called acute necrotizing ulcerative gingivitis (Trench mouth, or Vincent's gingivitis). Factors that can contribute to the development of this condition include abnormal dietary habits, hormonal changes, and emotional stress. Symptoms of gingivitis include red, swollen, and tender gums, bad breath, and poor taste in the mouth. Accompanying these problems is a significant loss of appetite, fever, and weakness. Chances of bacterial invasion are increased, thereby predisposing the patient to periodontitis.

Periodontitis: *Inflammation of the tissue that supports the teeth, usually resulting from progressive gingivitis.*

Management of these conditions requires good oral hygiene measures and modifications in the diet. Use of a pain–relieving mouthwash before eating may be helpful. Intake of fermentable carbohydrates such as simple sugars should be reduced significantly. A high–protein, high–calorie liquid diet should be given until tissue health is restored. This is followed by progression to a soft diet as tolerated. Spicy and acidic foods should be avoided because these are not well tolerated. Supplemental vitamins or minerals may be recommended.

In summary, nutrition plays a very crucial role in the clinical management of symptoms related to oral and gastrointestinal complications in the HIV–infected or AIDS patient. However, in situations where oral lesions are accompanied by marked reduction in appetite, fever, severe and uncontrolled diarrhea, and malabsorption, then regular feeding may not be adequate. In such cases, alternate forms of nutrition support may become necessary.

VI. ALTERNATE FORMS OF NUTRITION SUPPORT

Before designing an appropriate form of nutritional support for the AIDS patient, a thorough nutritional assessment of each patient is needed. This includes evaluation of diet; anthropometric measurements, laboratory values such as serum albumin, prealbumin, retinol–binding protein (protein that transports vitamin A), transferrin (protein that transports iron), etc., and psychosocial factors.

Anthropometric measurements: *Measurement of the height, weight, and proportions of the human body.*

A history of medications/drugs, etc. should also be collected because several of these affect the nutritional status (refer to Chapter 5).

Once all these data are collected, they are analyzed by a dietitian, and an individualized nutritional care prescription is devised based on the patient's needs. An enteral or parenteral form of nutritional support can be selected.

A. ENTERAL NUTRITION

Enteral nutrition: *Direct delivery of nutrients into the stomach, duodenum, or jejunum.*

When the patient needs some additional nutrients, defined formula diets that contain carbohydrate, protein, and fat can be given. In cases of severe oral lesions when feeding by mouth becomes practically impossible, a nasoenteric route of feeding can be employed. Blenderized feeding can be helpful in patients with esophagitis or esophageal ulceration.

Nasoenteric feeding: *Feeding through the nasal passage into the stomach, duodenum, or jejunum.*

Parenteral nutrition: *Direct delivery of nutrients into the blood circulation; can be complete and total or partial and supplemental; nutrients delivered by peripheral or central vein.*

B. PARENTERAL NUTRITION

When the patient is not able to tolerate adequate nutrients by the enteral route, parenteral nutrition may become necessary. Depending on the extent of the need, partial or complete parenteral nutrition should be used; however, this type of nutritional support should not be used for more than 10 days. Enteral and oral feeding should be resumed as soon as possible.

VII. SUMMARY

Management of oral and esophageal complications in the HIV–infected or AIDS patient represents a complex challenge to the caregivers or health professionals. To maintain adequate nutrition, selective and high–nutrient foods along with modified feeding techniques may become necessary. With adequate planning by the caregiver and cooperative support of the patient, optimum nutrition is possible. In the case of the HIV–infected or AIDS patient, optimum nutrition coupled with a positive life–style translates into enhanced quality of life.

REFERENCES

1. **Crocker, K. S.,** Gastrointestinal manifestations of the acquired immunodeficiency syndrome, *Nursing Clin. N. Am.,* 24, 395, 1989.
2. **Greenspan, D. and Greenspan, J. S.,** The oral clinical features of HIV infection, *Gastroenterol. Clin. N. Am.,* 17, 535, 1988.
3. **Barr, C. E. and Torosian, J. P.,** Oral manifestations in patients with AIDS or AIDS–related complex, *Lancet,* 2, 288, 1986.
4. **Walsh, T. J. and Pizzo, P. A.,** Nosocomial fungal infections, *Ann. Rev. Microbiol.,* 42, 517, 1988.
5. **McQuiggan, M. and Andrassy, R. S.,** Nutrition support of the AIDS patient, *(Sandoz Nutrition newsletter)* 10, 1, 1990.
6. **Volpe, F., Schwimmer, A., and Barr, C.,** Oral manifestation of disseminated *Mycobacterium avium-intracellulare* in a patient with AIDS, *Oral Surgery,* 60, 567, 1985.
7. Task Force on Nutrition Support in AIDS, Guidelines for nutrition support in AIDS, *Nutrition,* 5(1), 39, 1989.

Chapter 5

DRUG–INDUCED NUTRITIONAL COMPLICATIONS AND THEIR MANAGEMENT

Saroj Bahl

CONTENTS

I. INTRODUCTION

Prevention, treatment, and possibly a cure for AIDS will remain critical issues confronting health care professionals during the 1990s. It has been predicted that nearly 100% of the estimated 12 million HIV–positive persons will eventually develop AIDS. It has also been theorized that the progression of HIV infection to AIDS occurs despite any form of currently accepted therapy. The search for new curative drugs or those that can prevent or slow the growth of the virus is ongoing. During the period from 1987 to 1990, the attention of both clinicians and policymakers has shifted to early intervention in HIV illness because it is believed that a combination of drugs may be effective in retarding the progression of HIV infection to AIDS.[1] While all these drugs are very beneficial and used for a well–defined purpose, most of them seem to be associated with undesirable side effects as well. This chapter will focus on various types of drugs used in the clinical management of AIDS, their purpose in the treatment strategy, their adverse side effects, and the appropriate nutritional interventions that may become necessary.

II. GENERAL OBJECTIVES OF THERAPY

No single philosophy of treatment is agreed on when it comes to treatment of HIV infection or AIDS. The cornerstone of successful intervention is comprehensive inclusion — doing all of the things that make sense. General objectives of therapy include the delay in progression of HIV infection and maintenance of immune function.

A. COMPREHENSIVE TREATMENT STRATEGY

A comprehensive treatment strategy could include the use of several drugs such as antiviral medicines, immune modulators, and those that can prevent opportunistic infections, particularly Pneumocystis carinii pneumonia (PCP). The organism that causes PCP is widely prevalent in the environment but only becomes destructive in immunocompromised individuals, such as those suffering from HIV infection. A high percentage of individuals suffering from HIV–related illness succumb to PCP infection. Hence, PCP prophylaxis should form an integral component of the therapeutic regimen for HIV infection.

Immune Modulators: *Pharmaceuticals or drugs that help to increase the number of CD4 cells (cells that help in fighting infections) and restore immune function.*

B. MAINTENANCE OF GENERAL HEALTH

A strategy for maintenance of general health that combines adequate nutrition, rest, stress management, and avoidance of alcohol, smoking, and drugs should be emphasized (Figure 1). Many authorities emphasize the concepts of holistic health, which can include supportive therapies such as yoga, relaxation techniques, natural medicines, massage, spiritual support, and many others. While these strategies should not be used to replace the traditionally accepted therapeutic modalities, they may serve an important role as complementary approaches.

III. TREATMENT: WHEN SHOULD IT BEGIN?

There is a general agreement that in any serious illness, therapeutic interventions should be initiated as early as possible — usually right after the diagnosis is made. HIV–related illness is a serious life–threatening disease; hence, early intervention becomes even more essential. There is a debate, however, on the issue of timing of treatment with antiviral drugs, immune modulators, and medicines that prevent opportunistic infections.

Proponents of early intervention believe that antiviral medications can retard the progression of HIV infection. It is well accepted that HIV resists the attack of B cell antibodies and invades the T–4 or helper cells (see Chapter 1). This invasion leads to a chronic decline in the number of T–4 or CD4 cells.

Opponents of early intervention contend that HIV infection appears to be dormant for a long time, and they feel that it is futile to treat an inactive infection. The strong side effects associated with the use of antiviral medications are also a legitimate concern.

Recent studies with azidothymidine (zidovudine), however, indicate that early treatment appears to slow the progression toward AIDS and that side effects are minimal or virtually nonexistent in healthier patients. Hence, evidence seems to be heavily in favor of early intervention.

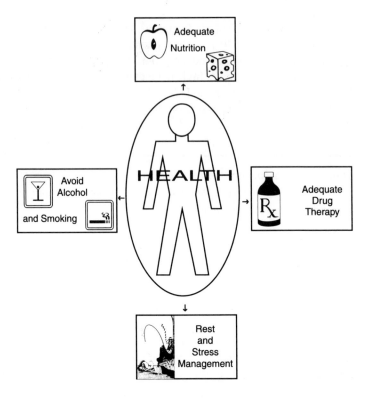

FIGURE 1.   Factors that contribute to maintenance of good health.

IV. STRATEGIES TO SLOW HIV INFECTION

Since 1985, it has been recognized that multiple therapies combining several drugs are more effective in the management of HIV infection than any single drug alone. A similar therapeutic approach has been shown to be effective in the treatment of other life–threatening diseases such as acute lymphocytic leukemia. Experiments with the treatment of such diseases have taught clinicians that combinations of drugs are more promising than single drugs.

A. COMBINATION THERAPY

Combination therapy utilizes drugs that act synergistically. This implies that one drug augments the action of the other, thereby producing a net effect that is together greater than the summative action of both drugs. For example, the action of the antiviral drug AZT is increased if it is combined with dideoxyinosine (ddI; Videx) or dideoxycytidine (ddC; HIVID). In general, an effective combination is one which combines drugs that are individually active to some degree, are known to act synergistically, and have different (rather than similar) side effects.

1. Goals of Combination Therapy

The goals of combination therapy thus include increased duration and extension of effectiveness of the treatments, diminution or elimination of resistant strains of the virus, and reduction of side effects associated with individual drugs. When used in combination, dosages of individual drugs can be reduced, thus minimizing the possibility of toxicity; however, the use of combination drugs is limited by the availability of drugs. The search for new, effective, and safe drugs is ongoing. Current research supports the combination of antiviral drugs with immunomodulating drugs. Human testing has been limited to AZT plus interferon, AZT plus interleukin, granulocyte macrophage-colony stimulating factor and AZT plus (GM–CSF). More recently, other combinations such as AZT and ddI or AZT and ddC have been tested. Results of these studies have not been very successful due to lack of available immune modulators. It also needs to be noted that all of these combination strategies include a single antiviral drug, which is AZT. As new drugs become available, other combinations with multiple antivirals and immune modulators will need to be tested. At present, several drugs fall into the category of "investigational new drugs" (INDs) and are not approved for sale. These can be legally obtained only by participating in controlled clinical trials. Marketing of such drugs is only permitted after they have been granted "new drug approval" (NDA) status.

2. Current Approach

In summary, it can be stated that three types of drugs/pharmaceuticals are used currently for the treatment of HIV infection in the early stages. These include antiviral medications, immune modulators, and those drugs that are used for the prevention or treatment of opportunistic infections. The last category can include a wide variety of drugs that may be used for the treatment of specific infections such as those caused by fungal, viral, bacterial, and protozoan agents. These opportunistic infections, which occur primarily in HIV–infected individuals, need to be prevented or treated as they occur. Major drugs, their purpose, their mode of action, and their significant side effects are summarized in Table 1.

B. ANTIVIRAL MEDICATIONS

1. Zidovudine (AZT)

AZT is the most widely used antiviral medication. Its purpose is to retard the replication of HIV, the virus that leads to AIDS. The virus requires an enzyme "reverse transcriptase" to be able to reproduce itself. AZT stops or slows the production of this enzyme, thereby preventing further viral reproduction. Nevertheless, AZT cannot kill infected cells and cannot remove the virus from them.

Several studies have supported the effectiveness of AZT; however, it is also believed that the benefits of the drug decrease over time. There are also some side effects associated with the drug. Common problems are anemia and decreased white blood cell counts, possibly due to bone marrow suppression

TABLE 1
Major Drugs Used in the Clinical Management of HIV Infection
(Early Stages)

Drug	Purpose	Mode of action	Significant side effects
ANTIVIRALS			
AZT (zidovudine)	Slows the reproduction of HIV	Stops or slows the production of reverse transcriptase, an enzyme that is required for reproduction of the virus	Anemia; reduced white blood cell counts, possibly due to bone marrow toxicity; pancreatitis (at higher doses); fat malabsorption
ddI (dideoxyinosine)	Slows the progression of HIV infection	Prevents the reproduction of HIV (by incorporation into viral DNA leading to inhibition of replication)	Pancreatitis (in susceptible candidates) and peripheral neuropathy (tingling sensation in hands/feet)
ddC (dideoxycytidine)	Slows the progression of HIV infection; improves the immune system	Suppresses the production of reverse transcriptase, an enzyme required for replication of the virus	Peripheral neuropathy (tingling sensation in the hands/feet)
Acyclovir (Zovirax®)	Treatment of several viral infections, such as cytomegalovirus, shingles, etc.	Slows the growth of the virus by inhibiting its reproduction; strengthens action of AZT	Nausea, vomiting, diarrhea, anorexia, headaches
IMMUNE MODULATORS			
Interferon (alpha 2A/2B) Interferon (beta) Interferon (gamma)	Regulation of immune system	Increases the number of functional CD4 cells; diminishes the autoimmune activities	Nausea, anorexia, taste alterations, fever, herpetic/non-herpetic eruptions
GM–CSF (granulocyte macrophage-colony stimulating factor)	Regulation of immune system	Increases the number of functional CD4 cells	No side effects reported

and toxicity. A reduction in the AZT dose may be helpful in decreasing some of these side effects.

2. Dideoxyinosine (ddI)

This is a new antiviral drug that slows or inhibits the reproduction of HIV. Hence, it is similar in action to AZT. Both drugs can cross the blood–brain barrier and act by inhibiting the ability of HIV–infected cells to produce new viruses. However, none of these drugs can eliminate or eradicate the infection.

One of the significant advantages that ddI has over AZT is that there are fewer side effects associated with its use. *In vitro* studies indicate that ddI prevents the reproduction of HIV but does not cause bone marrow toxicity. Anemia and suppression of white blood cells, which occur with AZT use, are not associated with administration of ddI; however, with higher doses, peripheral neuropathy and pancreatitis have been reported.

Peripheral neuropathy: *Painful nerve damage in the feet, characterized by tingling sensation in hands and feet.*

Pancreatitis: *Inflammation/irritation of the pancreatic tissue, characterized by abdominal pain, malabsorption of fat, diarrhea, etc.*

---

3. Dideoxycytidine (ddC)

This antiviral drug is in the same family as AZT and ddI. Its purpose in the therapy and mode of action is also fairly similar to AZT and ddI, i.e., it slows or stops the progression of HIV infection to AIDS. However, ddC cannot penetrate the blood–brain barrier as well as AZT can, so AZT may be a more effective drug to combat symptoms of HIV dementia.

HIV dementia: *Mental deterioration caused by central nervous system damage resulting from HIV infection.*

Studies indicate that the potential for ddC lies in its use as a combination drug with AZT. Patients who are on long–term AZT therapy can develop drug resistance; in those situations ddC is helpful. Incidence of side effects is low, particularly when the drug is used in combination with AZT. Also, it needs to be noted that ddC is given in extremely small doses, usually measured in fractions of milligrams.

Side effects associated with ddC include rashes, chest pain, mouth sores, fever, and nausea. More serious side effects are similar to ddI, i.e., peripheral neuropathy and pancreatitis (in susceptible individuals). Several studies are currently in progress to evaluate the efficacy of ddC in clinical management of HIV infection.

4. Acyclovir

This antiviral drug is primarily used for the treatment of herpes simplex infections. Some researchers have speculated that acyclovir may work synergistically with AZT by enhancing its effect, thereby permitting lower doses of AZT than commonly used. Further experimental trials are required to evaluate the combined effectiveness of AZT and acyclovir.

At present, acyclovir can be used as a preventive measure against herpes simplex, cytomegalovirus, Epstein–Barr virus, shingles, and hairy leukoplakia infections. Cytomegalovirus can cause serious infections in advanced stage of AIDS. Blindness can result from untreated cytomegalovirus retinitis. Hence, preventive or prophylactic treatment against this virus are recommended. Side effects are seldom observed. A few patients have reported nausea, vomiting, headaches, diarrhea, dizziness, and fatigue; however, these side effects are quite uncommon at standard and low doses.

C. IMMUNE MODULATORS

The general purpose of these drugs is to increase the number of functional CD4 cells and to restore the health of the immune system. Progression of HIV infection is sometimes accompanied by autoimmune effects; that is, the immune system begins attacking itself, leading to destruction of healthy cells along with infected ones. Immune modulators can assist in diminishing these autoimmune activities. Preliminary studies indicate that some drugs such as interferon (alpha, beta, and gamma), and GM–CSF may be of some value in increasing CD4 counts in HIV–infected individuals. Further research, however, is necessary to evaluate the efficacy of these drugs either alone or in combination with antiviral drugs such as AZT.

V. PREVENTION AND TREATMENT OF OPPORTUNISTIC INFECTIONS: VARIOUS DRUGS USED

Prevention and adequate treatment of the various opportunistic infections that are likely to occur in the HIV–infected patients can go a long way toward enhancing the longevity and quality of life in these individuals. Several drugs are used for this purpose; the drugs used for the treatment of some common opportunistic infections in HIV–infected individuals are summarized in Table 2.

Diagnosis of opportunistic infections is often difficult and needs to be confirmed. Several symptoms can have multiple causes. For example, diarrhea

TABLE 2
Drugs Used in the Clinical Management of Opportunistic Infections

Infections	Drugs used	Significant side effects
VIRAL		
Cytomegalovirus (CMV)	DHPG (dihydroxy–phenoxymethylguanine); ganciclovir	Thrombocytopenia, neutropenia, fever, rash, anemia
Herpes simplex and zoster	Acyclovir	Nausea, vomiting, anorexia
	Trifluorothymidine (topical solution)	Transient burning and stinging
BACTERIAL		
Mycobacterium tuberculosis and *M. avium* complex (MAC or MAI)	Isoniazid	Nausea, vomiting, dry mouth, fever, deficiencies of pyridoxine and niacin, peripheral neuropathy, and liver toxicity
	Pyrazinamide	Anorexia, fever, nausea, vomiting, liver toxicity (hepatitis), hemolytic anemia
	Rifampin	Rash, discoloration of body fluids, kidney and liver toxicity
FUNGAL		
Candidiasis (Thrush)	Ketoconazole	Headache, dizziness, drowsiness, liver toxicity
	Nystatin	Diarrhea, gastrointestinal upsets (with high doses)
	Fluconazole	Nausea, abdominal pain, headache, liver reactions (rarely)
Cryptococcosis	Amphotericin B	Chills, fever, headache, anemia, vomiting diarrhea, metallic taste, hypokalemia (lowered potassium in blood) and hypomagnesemia (lowered magnesium in blood), lowered blood presure, abnormal heart beat
	Fluconazole	Same as above
Histoplasmosis	Amphotericin B; Fluconazole	Same as above
PROTOZOAL		
Toxoplasma gondii (toxoplasmosis)	Pyrimethamine	Nausea/vomiting, anorexia, glossitis (tongue tenderness), anemia (megaloblastic — large cells), taste alterations

TABLE 2 (continued)
Drugs Used in the Clinical Management of Opportunistic Infections

Infections	Drugs used	Significant side effects
Cryptosporidiosis	Paromomycin (Humatin)	Nausea, hearing loss, kidney toxicity, vomiting, colitis
Pneumocystis carinii pneumonia (PCP)	Pentamidine (given intravenously)	Nausea, vomiting, taste alterations, lowered glucose and calcium in blood, (sometimes elevated blood glucose)
	Dapsone	Anorexia, vomiting, nausea, anemia (with deficiency of the enzyme glucose-6-phosphate dehydrogenase)
	Bactrim™	Rash, fever, anemia, nausea, suppression of white blood cells, liver irritation

can be caused by a number of infectious agents including cryptosporidiosis and cytomegalovirus (CMV) colitis. Not all HIV–infected individuals experience the same symptoms. Some other symptoms may be rare or possibly can be confused with drug–related effects.

Treatment strategies and dosage levels of medications are controversial. These have to be adjusted for the individual needs of each patient. Every person has a different immune status and medical history; therapeutic modalities that are appropriate for some may not be adequate for others. It also needs to be noted that experiments on various drugs and their efficacy are being conducted all over the world, and the existing data related to some drugs are based on limited observations.

A. PNEUMOCYSTIS CARINII PNEUMONIA (PCP) PROPHYLAXIS

When CD4 counts fall below 200 in HIV-seropositive patients, it is essential to implement PCP prophylaxis. PCP is a lung infection that occurs rarely in the general population; however, it constitutes the leading cause of death in HIV–infected individuals. This infection can be prevented with adequate prophylaxis.

One of the most popular and effective forms of PCP prophylaxis is aerosolized pentamidine. This approach, which involves administration of aerosol pentamidine into the patient's lungs by a respiratory therapist, is promising and has minimal side effects because the drug is not circulated throughout the body. However, it is expensive ($59 to $125 per treatment), inconvenient, and not available everywhere. Also, its long–term efficacy is questionable. As a result, many physicians are recommending oral doses of trimethoprim/sulfamethoxazole (Bactrim™ or Septra®) and dapsone, both of which prevent or retard PCP by inhibiting microbial growth. Side effects associated with the administration of these drugs include nausea, vomiting, fever, rash, and lowered white and red blood cell count.

While some physicians support prophylactic treatment for certain opportunistic infections, others do not. Proponents of prophylaxis argue that it is desirable to prevent an active infection that may also stimulate the immune system causing increased replication of HIV. Also, in cases of infections such as PCP, relapses can be very difficult. Opponents of prophylaxis for opportunistic infections maintain that resistance to treatments may occur and that available evidence to support such strategies is insufficient.

Prophylaxis: *Avoidance of disease by using preventive treatments such as drugs, etc.*

B. VIRAL INFECTIONS

Cytomegalovirus is a serious viral infection that can affect the esophagus (gullet) and colon, resulting in inflammation and ulceration. In rare cases, pneumonia may occur; in its serious form, CMV can lead to retinitis and blindness. This infection is treated by ganciclovir (dihydroxyphenoxy–methylguanine or DHPG). Side effects associated with its usage include thrombocytopenia, neutropenia, fever, and rash.

Thrombocytopenia: *Decrease in the number of platelets.*

Neutropenia: *Decrease in the number of neutrophilic leukocytes in the blood.*

Herpes simplex and zoster are viral infections that can lead to painful blisters, ulcers, itching on the lips, anus and/or genitals. Treatment is with acyclovir (Zovirax®) given orally or intravenously. Associated side effects with its usage include nausea, vomiting, and anorexia.

C. BACTERIAL INFECTIONS

HIV–infected individuals are very prone to developing tuberculosis, caused by *Mycobacterium tuberculosis* as well as another similar infection caused by *Mycobacterium avium* complex (MAC). Both infections have similar symptoms that include persistent fever, night sweats, abdominal pain, weakness, dizziness, and nausea. Tuberculosis may be pulmonary, which involves the lungs, or extrapulmonary, which may affect other organs. Swollen lymph glands are observed in both these bacterial infections. There is no widely accepted, standard treatment for the clinical management of these infections. A combination of drugs including isoniazid, pyrazinamide, and rifampin can be used. Usage of these drugs is accompanied by several side effects ranging from mild effects such as nausea, vomiting, and fever to more serious threats such as liver and kidney toxicity.

D. FUNGAL INFECTIONS

Candidiasis, a fungal infection, is very common in HIV–infected individuals. This condition is characterized by white patches on gums and tongue or its lining. The esophagus may get affected, leading to difficulty in eating. Treatment of this fungal infection is with several drugs — ketoconazole, nystatin, and fluconazole. Side effects associated with these drugs include nausea, headache, and gastrointestinal upsets. Liver toxicity has been reported with the usage of ketoconazole.

Cryptococcal disease (or cryptococcosis) is another fungal infection that may involve several organs, including the brain (meningitis), lungs (pneumonia), and multiple other organs (disseminated infection). Treatment is with amphotericin B and fluconazole. Side effects associated with this therapy include diarrhea, vomiting, fever, and anemia. Lowered magnesium and potassium levels in the blood also have been reported. The same therapy is used for the treatment of histoplasmosis, a fungal infection characterized by weight loss, skin lesions, lymphadenopathy, difficult breathing, and anemia.

Lymphadenopathy: *Swollen lymph nodes or a disease of lymph nodes.*

E. PROTOZOAL INFECTIONS

Protozoal infections that may occur in HIV–infected individuals include *Toxoplasma gondii,* (toxoplasmosis) cryptosporidiosis, and Pneumocystis carinii pneumonia. Toxoplasmosis is a serious infection characterized by encephalitis, altered mental state (lethargy, confusion, etc.), paralysis, seizures, severe headaches, fever, and coma. Treatment is with the drug, pyrimethamine. Side effects of this drug include nausea, vomiting, anorexia, anemia, and taste alterations.

Encephalitis: *Inflammation of the brain.*

Cryptosporidiosis is a protozoal infection that is characterized primarily by diarrhea (with frequent watery stools). Other symptoms include nausea, abdominal cramping, flatulence, weight loss, and loss of appetite. Serious consequences such as fluid and electrolyte imbalances and dehydration may follow. While there is no standard treatment for this infection, a combination of drugs such as paromomycin (Humatin), spiramycin, and fluconazole has been used. Side effects associated with the use of these drugs range from nausea and vomiting to kidney toxicity and hearing loss.

Treatment of PCP, which has been discussed before, is similar to its prophylaxis. Drugs such as dapsone and Bactrim™ can be administered orally. Side effects of these drugs include fever, rash, nausea, and anemia. Other significant effects include lowered red and white blood cell count as well as liver inflammation.

VI. SUMMARY OF SIGNIFICANT SIDE EFFECTS ASSOCIATED WITH DRUG THERAPY

Table 3 presents a summary of the significant side effects that are associated with drugs commonly used in HIV–infected individuals. These effects have been categorized according to various body systems or organs. As is clear from perusal of this listing, the effects vary from somewhat minor consequences such as nausea and vomiting to quite serious ones such as liver and kidney toxicity. Because some of these effects occur with prolonged usage of the drug, some of the side effects can be minimized with adjustments in dosage, timing, and schedule. With other side effects such as anemia associated with AZT and several other medications, some other drugs such as erythropoietin (EPO) can be used.

Various nutritional strategies and some simple dietary modifications can help alleviate minor problems such as nausea, vomiting, dry mouth, taste alterations, etc. Nutrition can perform a very crucial role in the management of several side effects. Nutritional interventions designed to alleviate drug–induced effects are summarized in Table 4.

VII. NUTRITIONAL MANAGEMENT OF SIGNIFICANT PROBLEMS ASSOCIATED WITH DRUG THERAPY

A. WEIGHT LOSS
The primary causes of malnutrition and the attendant loss of lean body mass/weight loss are reduced food intake, hypermetabolism, and malabsorption. Several drugs such as isoniazid, nystatin, octreotide, and others are associated with malabsorption of nutrients. Nutritional management consists of provision of an adequate amount of calories, protein, vitamins, and minerals through well–planned, nutritious, and palatable meals. However, when nutritional needs cannot be met with oral feeding alone, administration of high–calorie, high–protein supplements becomes necessary. Small meals or frequent snacks of protein and calorie–dense foods (e.g., eggs, cheese, instant breakfast drinks, ice cream, custard, etc.) may be helpful in preventing weight loss (Figure 2).

TABLE 3
A Summary of Significant Side Effects
that Are Associated with Drug Therapy

Body system organ	Effects
General	Fever
	Weight loss
	Poor appetite
	Headache
	Dizziness
	Drowsiness
Gastrointestinal	Nausea
	Vomiting
	Diarrhea
	Taste alterations
	Dry mouth (xerostomia)
	Inflammation of the tongue (glossitis)
	Inflammation of colon (colitis)
Circulatory system/blood	Anemia
	Hemolytic anemia
	Reduced white blood cell count (leukocytopenia)
	Reduced number of platelets in blood (thrombocytopenia)
	Reduced number of neutrophils in blood (neutropenia)
	Low magnesium in blood (hypomagnesemia)
	Hypo– and hyperglycemia
	Low potassium in blood (hypokalemia)
	Blood pressure changes
Specific organs	Liver enlargement, inflammation (hepatitis)
	Inflammation of pancreas (pancreatitis)
	Kidney dysfunction/toxicity
Nervous system	Tingling sensation in hands and feet (peripheral neuropathy)
	Headache
Skin	Rash
	Herpetic eruptions

B. PROBLEMS ASSOCIATED WITH GASTROINTESTINAL TRACT

1. Nausea/Vomiting

Nausea and vomiting may appear to be relatively minor problems; however, they can significantly compromise food intake and lead to weight loss and malnutrition. Nutritional management consists of consumption of

TABLE 4
Nutritional Management of Significant Problems
Associated with Drug Therapy

Problem	Nutritional management strategies
Weight loss	Use small meals or frequent snacks Use high–calorie, high–protein supplements such as cheese, milk shakes, ice cream, custard, etc. Monitor weight regularly
Nausea/vomiting	Frequent, small meals rather than three large ones Offer soft, bland foods, low in fat
Diarrhea	Restrict fatty foods and lactose–containing foods Increase intake of carbonated beverages, high-potassium foods (bananas, mangoes, etc.) Eat low–fiber, low–fat foods, e.g., white rice, bread, cooked fruits such as applesauce, etc.
Taste alterations/dry mouth (xerostomia)	Use saliva stimulants such as sour candy/gum Use well–seasoned foods and fruit-flavored supplements Avoid red meat, chocolate, coffee, and tea
Inflammation of tongue and mouth (glossitis and stomatitis)	Avoid acidic, spicy foods or other irritants Soft, bland foods may be better tolerated High–calorie, high–protein supplements may be given if food intake remains low
Inflammation of colon (colitis)	Use a low–fat, low–residue diet Avoid or restrict lactose–rich foods Avoid caffeine Small, frequent meals
Anemia	Use iron–rich and folate–rich foods Blood transfusions may become necessary in severe cases
Hyperglycemia and hypoglycemia	Plan a diet according to guidelines established by the American Dietetic Association Consume regular meals and snacks
Organ toxicities (liver, kidney, pancreas)	Supportive nutritional therapy including adequate calories, protein, and vitamin-mineral supplements In chronic pancreatitis, pancreatic enzymes may need to be administered with each meal or snack

small, frequent meals throughout the day rather than three large meals (Figure 3). Large meals tend to cause abdominal distention, which further aggravates the nausea. Soft and bland foods that are low in fat are generally well tolerated.

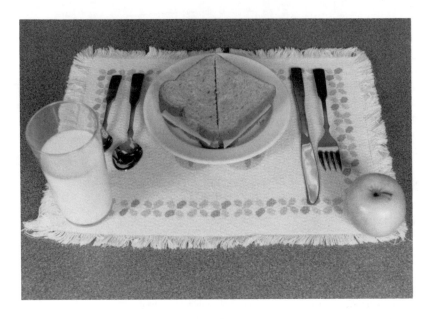

FIGURE 2. Frequent snacks of protein and calorie–dense foods, e.g., cheese sandwiches and instant drinks, may be helpful in preventing weight loss.

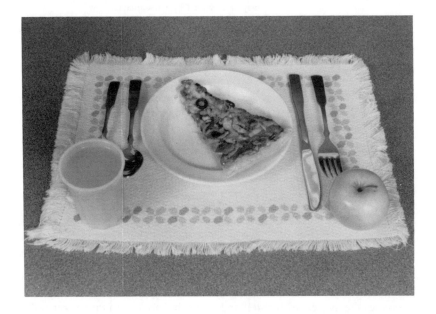

FIGURE 3. Small meals offered frequently are generally better tolerated by the AIDS patient.

2. Diarrhea

Diarrhea is caused by several opportunistic pathogens in HIV–infected individuals; it may also be associated with the use of several drugs. Detailed management of this problem is discussed in Chapter 3. Osmotic diarrhea is associated with water and potassium depletion. Patients with this type of diarrhea and a less severe form of malabsorption may benefit from bowel rest, antidiarrheal agents, albumin replacement therapy, and some dietary modifications. Modifications in dietary strategies may include restriction of lactose–containing and fatty foods, increase of fluid and electrolyte intake (carbonated and/or electrolyte repletion beverages, bananas, or mangoes), and use of low–fat, low–fiber foods such as white rice, white bread, and cooked fruits and vegetables. Diarrhea of a secretory origin does not respond to dietary interventions or to withholding food. This type of diarrhea generally results from infectious enteropathogens and hence should be treated accordingly.

3. Taste Alterations/Dry Mouth (Xerostomia)

Several drugs such as pentamidine, acyclovir, azidothymidine (AZT), and amphotericin B can cause dysgeusia or taste alterations. Other drugs that are used for topical application such as tetracycline suspensions and chlorhexidine gluconate (Peridex®) may also lead to taste alterations. These distortions can vary from loss of taste, or abnormal taste to "metallic" taste sensations. Several of these taste changes are accompanied by a dry mouth (xerostomia) as well. Nutritional strategies that may assist in the management of these problems include the use of saliva stimulants such as sour candy, a regular diet with many cold foods, well–seasoned foods as tolerated, and fruit–flavored supplements. Some foods such as chocolate, coffee, tea, and red meats may be poorly tolerated and hence should be avoided (see Chapter 4 for treatment of xerostomia).

4. Inflammation of the Tongue (Glossitis) and Mouth Area (Stomatitis)

Certain drugs such as AZT, trimethoprim/sulfamethoxazole, trimetrexate, and bleomycin sulfate are associated with ulcers and inflammation of the mouth area. In such cases, acidic, citrus foods and extremes of temperature in serving food should be avoided. Spicy foods should also be limited or avoided. If food intake remains low, then intermittent or continuous nutritional support such as high–calorie, high–protein supplements should be administered (see Chapter 4).

5. Inflammation of the Colon (Colitis)

Acute colitis, or inflammation of the colon, is associated with certain drugs such as spiramycin, which is used for the treatment of cryptosporidiosis (a protozoal infection). Nutritional management of colitis may involve a low–fat, low–residue, low–lactose, and caffeine–free diet. Small, frequent meals may be better tolerated than three large ones.

C. PROBLEMS ASSOCIATED WITH BLOOD CHEMISTRY
1. Anemia
The use of several drugs such as azidothymidine (AZT), foscarnet, dapsone, and pyrimethamine is associated with anemia. This condition needs to be carefully evaluated before institution of therapy. Anemia may be the microcytic type (small red blood cells) or the megaloblastic type (large red blood cells). Both of these are caused by different factors, so the treatment/therapy needs to be selected accordingly. Nutritional management strategies include an increased intake of iron–rich foods and iron supplements for microcytic anemia and liberal consumption of folate–rich foods or folate supplements for megaloblastic anemia. In severe cases of anemia, a blood transfusion may become necessary.

2. Hyperglycemia and Hypoglycemia
The use of pentamidine and certain other drugs is accompanied with alterations in glucose tolerance resulting in hyperglycemia (elevated glucose levels in blood) or hypoglycemia (diminished glucose in blood). Nutritional management of both of these problems is fairly similar and includes strategies such as consumption of regular meals and snacks and an individualized diet, principles of which have been established by the American Dietetic Association. In the case of hyperglycemia, insulin may need to be administered. Antihypoglycemic drugs may become necessary in the treatment of hypoglycemia.

D. ORGAN TOXICITIES: LIVER, KIDNEY, AND PANCREAS
Certain drugs such as pyrazinamide, amphotericin B, and foscarnet may cause damage to vital organs such as the liver, kidney, and pancreas. Some of these effects can be minimized by adjustments in the dosages of drugs, length of use, etc. When inflammation does occur, nutritional management can be (at the best) supportive rather than therapeutic. In the case of pancreatitis, the use of pancreatic enzymes at every meal may become necessary to facilitate normal digestion.

In addition to the side effects that have been discussed, several others ranging from mild effects such as headache, dizziness, and drowsiness to severe and serious ones such as renal dysfunction (abnormal kidney function) and neuropathies (abnormal nerve function) have been reported. Although there are no specific nutritional management strategies for these problems, maintenance of good nutrition may still be helpful in reducing their impact on general health. An individual who is in good health and has an adequate nutritional status prior to the initiation of drug therapy certainly has a better chance of withstanding the adverse effects associated with the therapeutic regimen.

E. NUTRIENT DEFICIENCIES
Deficiencies of some nutrients such as folate, pyridoxine, and vitamin B_{12} have been reported in HIV–infected individuals. These may result from various

opportunistic infections, the HIV infection itself, or the use of several drugs. It is also well known and accepted that many nutrient deficiencies are associated with suboptimal functioning of the immune system. Hence, a dietary prescription designed to include liberal amounts of all essential nutrients may be very helpful in improving the quality of life for the HIV–infected or AIDS patient. In addition, a well–nourished individual may increase his/her chances of experiencing minimal adverse effects associated with drug therapy.

VIII. SUMMARY

Management of HIV infection necessitates the use of several drugs. Although all these therapeutic medications are necessary and serve a very useful purpose, all of them are associated with side effects that may range from mild to severe. Some of these effects can be minimized with adjustments in dosages, treatment schedules, and combinations of drugs. However, many of these side effects may persist and affect the nutritional status of the patient. On the other hand, nutritional status can affect the tolerance of drug therapy, thus the role of nutrition in the therapeutic management of drug–related complications cannot be overemphasized. A nutritious diet that includes liberal amounts of all essential nutrients, as well as one that is presented in adequate consistency, texture and flavor, can go a long way in improving the quality of the HIV–

REFERENCES

1. **Arno, P. S., Shenson, D., Siegel, N. F., Franks, P., and Lee, P. R.,** Economic and policy implications of early intervention in HIV disease, *J. Am. Med. Assoc.,* 262, 1493, 1989.
2. Project information, treatment strategy, *Proj. Inf. Discuss. Pap.,* 1, 4, 1990.
3. Project information, combination therapy — why, how and when, *Proj. Inf. Perspec.,* 10, 3, 1991.
4. Project information, guide to opportunistic infections, *Proj. Inf. Perspect.,* 11, 11, 1991.
5. **Ghiron, L., Dwyer, J., and Stollman, L. B.,** Nutrition support of the HIV–positive, ARC and AIDS patient, *Clin. Nutr.,* 8, 103, 1989.
6. **Keithley, J. K. and Kohn, C. L.,** Managing nutritional problems in people with AIDS, *Oncol. Nursing Forum,* 17, 23, 1990.
7. Task Force on Nutrition Support in AIDS, Guidelines for nutrition support in AIDS, *Nutrition,* 5(1), 39, 1989.

Chapter 6

DEFENSIVE EATING

J. F. Hickson, Jr.

CONTENTS

I. INTRODUCTION

A. EATING DEFENSIVELY

Watch out for the other guy. That is the basic idea behind defensive driving. In eating, the same approach works very well for those who are infected with human immunodeficiency virus (HIV) and for those who are not. Watch out for food heavily contaminated with microorganisms.

All food is contaminated with microbes, but the microbial count becomes unsafe when food has been mishandled. Steer clear of food that might be heavily contaminated, because it can make a person very sick. Know what you are eating, where it came from, and how it was prepared.

Those who have control over their personal food supply system are unlikely to contract a foodborne illness. Happily, little change is needed in food preferences to accommodate the need for higher standards of food sanitation. Additionally, the guidelines for eating defensively for persons living with HIV are not any different than they would be for other immunocompromised persons including diabetics, elderly people, cancer patients, transplant recipients, pregnant women, and infants.

B. FOOD AS A VECTOR FOR DISEASE

There are many different kinds of microbes, but only certain ones present a problem in regard to food safety and sanitation. It is common to classify them into three types according to the system developed by the classical biologist Keeton[1] (Table 1). Accordingly, food microbes loosely termed as fungi include bacteria, yeasts, and molds.

Since microbes are present in or on all foods, it is a good rule to consider all products as being contaminated. Whether a food will make someone sick if eaten (i.e., food poisoning) depends on two things: (1) how many living cells are present on the food and (2) how many cells are needed to cause illness (virulence). Because food can serve as a vehicle for the transmission of disease–causing microbes from a source to the one eating it, it is said to be a "vector" for disease.

C. FOOD MICROBES AND OPPORTUNISTIC INFECTIONS

Immunocomprised persons are much more susceptible to food poisoning than healthy persons. Specifically, it takes fewer organisms to cause disease in persons with acquired immunodeficiency syndrome (AIDS), or PWAs. A microbe that is able to flourish in the body when it normally would not is termed "opportunistic". In PWAs, foodborne infections last longer, and recovery is slower. Compounding the problem, disease–causing microbes in the gastrointestinal (GI) canal are more likely to "jump" into the bloodstream due to the compromised integrity of the wall barrier. Then whole–body (systemic) infections result, and they can be resistant to treatment in PWAs. Most importantly, whole–body infections are often life threatening because the weak immune system of a PWA cannot check the activity of the invader. The microbe rapidly poisons the body, killing it.

D. USDA PERSPECTIVE ON IMMUNOCOMPROMISED PERSONS

The U.S. Department of Agriculture (USDA) recognizes that microbes are a natural, unavoidable part of life. They are present on the skin surface, in the GI tract, and in or on all foods. Although cleaning may remove visible dirt and debris, do not assume that the food is wholesome for consumption. Microbes

TABLE 1
Classification of Microorganisms According to the
System of Classical Biologist, W. T. Keeton

I. Animals
    A. Protozoans — single-cell animals
    B. Multicellular animals
II. Plants[a]
    A. Algae — contain chlorophyll (photosynthetic)
    B. Fungi — do not contain chlorophyll (nonphotosynthetic)
        1. Molds — multicellular-hyphae mass with or without cross walls
        2. Yeasts — single cells (spherical in shape: 2 to 7 microns[b] in diameter)
        3. Bacteria — single cells (rodlike in shape: 2 to 10 microns long, 0.5 to 2.5
           microns in diameter)

Source: From Keeton, W. T., *Biological Science,* 2nd ed., Norton, New York, 1972, chap. 21. With permission.

[a] Plants: Without true roots, stems, or leaves; [b] micron = 1/1,000,000 meter or about 0.000039 inch.

should be considered as an inherent defect of foods that does not require labeling.

Consumers must see themselves as taking part in the chain of responsibility for the sanitary quality of the food they eat. Other members of the chain include the farmer, industrial food processor, grocer, and restaurant operator. The government is limited in the extent to which it can monitor all the links of the chain; it cannot guarantee absolute safety at any point. Unfortunately, many believe that the government protects them against mishandling of food. This is unrealistic. Consumers have the ultimate responsibility for assuring the sanitary quality of their food.

E. THE RESPONSIBILITY FOR FOOD SAFETY ASSURANCE

Food undergoes many inspections before it reaches the shelves of the grocery store; however, no one can absolutely guarantee that food for sale is safe to eat from the standpoint of microbial content. Therefore, consumers must assume the responsibility as final inspectors of the food they purchase and eat.

Being final inspector means more than a cursory look at the food being purchased at the store. It also encompasses all of the things you need to do to protect food from becoming a breeding ground for disease–causing microbes, including care during transport, storage, preparation, and processing (i.e., cooking, etc.) in the home. The consumer is in full control during all of these critical stages.

It is a common misconception among American consumers that inspections by city, county, state, or federal officials are going to protect them from any exposure to microbes in foods. Some express a belief that food for sale in the grocery store is free of microbes altogether (sterile). However, there is no truth in this belief, since food is a natural vector for microbes. Governmental agencies seek only to prevent abuse of food that might lead to large–scale outbreaks of food poisoning. The prevention of small outbreaks at home is the consumer's problem; it is everyone's responsibility to know how to eat defensively.

II. NECESSARY CONDITIONS FOR MICROBES IN FOOD

Each food has its own internal "environment" which is the result of seven factors operating together including (1) amount of moisture, (2) water activity, (3) presence of oxygen, (4) temperature, (5) nutrient availability, (6) acidity, and (7) presence of naturally occurring or added growth inhibitors. The environment of any given food determines whether a particular microbe will find it harsh or favorable; not every microbe likes the same environment. Consequently, different expressions of the seven factors result in many dissimilar environments, each of which is favorable to some microbe.

A. MOISTURE
Water is essential for the growth of all microorganisms since it is the solvent in which chemical and biological reactions occur; this is a passive role of water. Additionally, water actually participates in certain reactions such as those resulting in the breakdown of complex food components, proteins, carbohydrates, and fats in the stomach and intestines. Water is present in fluid beverages and solid foods, including those that have been "dried" (Table 2).

Despite the presence of water in foods, there may be no evidence of microbial activity, but this does not mean that there are not any microbes present in or on the surface of a given food. Instead, it likely means that the amount of water is insufficient or one or more of the other six factors determining the food environment are not permitting microbial activity.

B. WATER ACTIVITY
Water present in foods is not always fully available for the use of microbes. Water that is not available is said to be "bound" to other food components, especially sugar, salt, and proteins; water that is available is termed "free". Therefore, it is not meaningful to discuss the susceptibility of foods to microbes in terms of water content alone. It is also necessary to consider how much of the water present can be used; this information is expressed in terms of a "water activity" score (Table 2).

The concept of water activity is used to express the relationship between free and bound water in a food. Water activity scores can be used to predict whether a food will allow the growth of a microbe and if so which type (bacteria, yeast, or mold). Each of the three types of fungi has a minimum water activity score (Table 3).

TABLE 2

Water Activity Scores[a] and
Percent Water Composition Data
For Selected Foods[6-8]

Food group	Water activity score	Water (%)
Fruits		
Dried, varieties	60–65	15
Fresh, varieties	97–100	80
Grain products		
Bread	70–80	36
Flour, all purpose	67–87	12
Dairy products		
Cheese, Brie	98	48
Cheese, cheddar	95	37
Cheese, cottage	99	79
Meat		
Meat, cured	87–95	58
Meat, fresh	95–100	64
Sweets		
Candy	70–75	8
Honey	60–65	17
Molasses	65–70	24

[a] Score system: 0 = lowest (no water available for microbial use); 100 = maximum (all water available).

TABLE 3

Minimum Water Activity Scores of Foods
Necessary for Activity of Each of the
Three Types of Fungi Found in Foods

Type of fungi	Minimum score	Spoilage pattern
Bacteria	90	Predominate over yeasts and molds
Yeasts	87	Predominate over molds
Molds	70	

Outside of its water activity range, a given type of microbe will not be active; however, there is an exception to this rule. The rule of "spoilage pattern" states that bacteria are dominant over yeasts and molds and yeasts are dominant over molds. For example, if meat has a water activity score of 95, then it is possible that all three types of fungi could be active on or in it. Nevertheless, this does not occur because bacteria can grow and reproduce faster than the other two types. Consequently, bacteria will take over the meat before yeast or mold can — they will be shut out.

A second exception is in regard to foods that are acidic such as tomatoes. Although there is a lot of water present in a tomato, bacteria and even yeasts will not be able to spoil it because these two types of fungi do not tolerate acid very well. Instead, only microbes that "love" acid will be able to survive and take over; the organisms that will spoil a tomato are molds.

C. OXYGEN

All microbes require oxygen in some form as an electron acceptor so that energy can be made from the breakdown of food materials. The ability to tolerate atmospheric oxygen is the basis for classification of microbes. In some cases, the oxygen in the air is suitable, and these organisms are "aerobic". Those that cannot tolerate the form of oxygen in the air are termed "anaerobic". A third category can tolerate atmospheric oxygen, but only in small amounts.

D. TEMPERATURE

Water is the solvent in which chemical and biological reactions occur for all living organisms, including microbes (Section II.A). This statement assumes that water is in the liquid state. If water is in the form of ice or steam, then the reactions of life cannot occur. Furthermore, considering water in the liquid form only, each microbe has an optimal temperature for maximum activity and minimum and a maximum temperatures for activity (Figure 1).

1. Cold–Loving Microorganisms

Microbes that love the cold are maximally active within the temperature range of 10 to 30°C (50 to 86°F), but they will grow in temperatures as low as 0°C (32°F, "freezing") (Figure 2). Therefore, just keeping a food in the refrigerator will not ensure that microbes will not spoil it or multiply, resulting in food poisoning. An excellent example is ground beef; it is usually contaminated with *Pseudomonas*. This microbe produces a slimy substance on the surface of meat after a few days depending on how old it was when purchased. The presence of this slime indicates an overwhelming presence of spoilage microbes on the meat, and it should be discarded. Meat that cannot be eaten immediately should always be frozen rock solid. Remember, if a freezer cannot freeze rock solid, then do not freeze in it because microbes will survive and grow, possibly leading to illness if not spoilage of the foods.

2. Pathogens and the Temperature Danger Zone

Many pathogens prefer temperatures similar to those of warm–blooded animals at 25 to 40°C (77 to 104°F). Since it is not a healthy idea to encourage the growth of these disease–causing microbes, it is important to keep food out

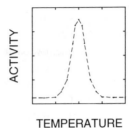

TEMPERATURE

FIGURE 1.   Nonspecific plot of the activity levels of most microbes found in foods at different food temperatures. Each microbe has an optimal temperature at which activity reaches a maximum; it is characteristic that activity decreases as temperature rises or falls from the optimum.

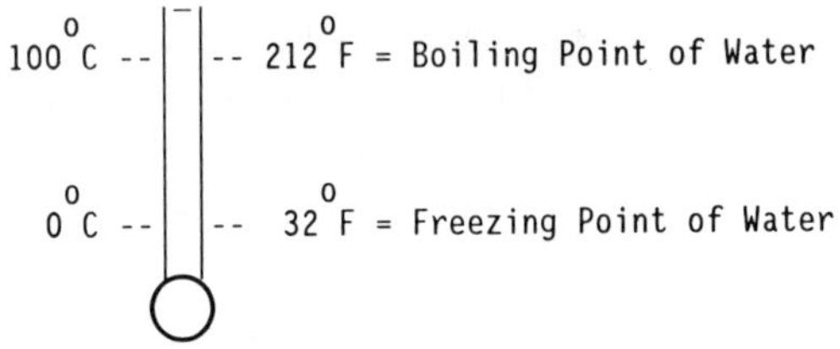

```
100°C  --  |  --  212°F  =  Boiling Point of Water


  0°C  --  |  --   32°F  =  Freezing Point of Water
```

FIGURE 2.   Thermometer with boiling and freezing points of water expressed in degrees Centigrade (°C) and Farenheit (°F).

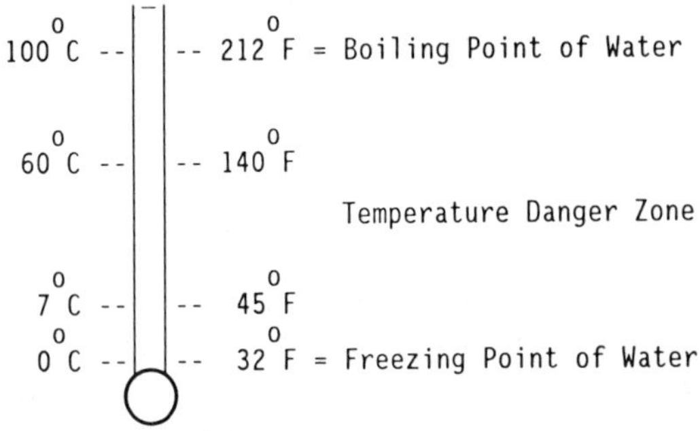

```
100°C  --  |  --  212°F  =  Boiling Point of Water


 60°C  --  |  --  140°F

                          Temperature Danger Zone


  7°C  --  |  --   45°F
  0°C  --  |  --   32°F  =  Freezing Point of Water
```

FIGURE 3.   Thermometer with the temperature danger zone identified between the boiling and freezing points of water.

of this "temperature danger zone" (Figure 3). Many persons become ill with food poisoning simply because they failed to keep cold foods cold and hot foods hot.

One of the most common problems is holding food at a "warm" temperature for too long after cooking. During this holding period, microbes find their way to the food and begin to grow and multiply. Bacteria can reproduce every 20 minutes under ideal circumstances. At that rate, a single cell can produce more

TABLE 4
Multiplication of Bacteria
Under Ideal Conditions

Elapsed time	Number of organisms
Begin	1
20 min	2
40 min	4
1 h	8
2 h	64
3 h	512
4 h	4,096
5 h	32,768
6 h	262,144
7 h	2,097,152
8 h	16,777,216

than two million cells within 8 hours (Table 4). Assuming there are many points of contamination of a food at the zero time, then it likely will become a disease vector within a practical period of only 4 to 8 hours.

3. Heat–Loving Microorganisms

At the high end of the scale are those microbes that prefer being in very warm to hot water, with temperatures ranging from 45 to 65°C (113 to 149°F). Some foods are served warm instead of hot; consequently, heat–loving microbes are still living in them. Fortunately, these survivors are not pathogens; they are spoilage–causing microbes.

For example, consider raw milk pasteurized using the modern "high–temperature, short–time" method; it is heated to a temperature of 72°C (162°F) for a minimum of 15 seconds. Despite this heat treatment, heat–loving microbes such as *Streptococcus* and *Lactobacillus* survive. They eventually spoil milk even if it is kept cold in the refrigerator; spoilage is observed with an acid taste and curdled appearance.

Another good example is canned food. Canned foods are usually only heated to destroy disease–causing organisms. Spoilage microbes remain, but they are dormant at the relatively cool temperatures of your kitchen. Canned food products could be heated to a higher temperature and/or for a longer period to render them sterile; however, the products suffer great loss of color and texture. Because it is not necessary and since quality would suffer greatly, canned foods are only heated sufficiently to kill pathogens, and these canned products are termed "commercially sterile".

E. NUTRIENT AVAILABILITY

In order for microbes to be active, they must find in their host foods a rich supply of nutrients to satisfy their own needs. These nutrients are the same as a person's needs (with certain exceptions), including minerals, water, proteins, ammonia, nitrates, vitamins, and energy (especially from sugars). Depending on which nutrients are available, the particular type of microbe to grow can be predicted. For example, if milk sugar — lactose — is present, then *Lactobacillus* will grow.

F. ACIDITY

Foods are loosely grouped in two categories according to how much acidity they contain (Table 5). Acidic foods, such as tomatoes, are called "high–acid" foods; those that are not acidic, such as corn, are termed "low–acid" foods. Acid has a practical importance in foods because bacteria only grow in low–acid foods. Yeasts grow in slightly acidic foods, right on the border between high– and low–acid foods. Molds will grow in foods ranging in acidity from high to low.

G. GROWTH INHIBITORS

These are compounds or barriers that interfere with the metabolism of the microbe so that it cannot be active in foods. These may be naturally occurring in foods or added by the processor (natural and synthetic preservatives). One of the most interesting examples of growth inhibitors is the shell of an egg which serves as a physical barrier to invading microbes. Close examination of the shell reveals that it is much more than a solid wall. The shell is more of a membrane with pores too small for microbes to breach, yet oxygen and carbon dioxide can move across it to allow the growing chick to survive.

Another growth inhibitor is sugar, which can be considered as a natural food additive in jelly, jams, and preserves. Sugar binds water to such an extent that it is not available to microbes present in the condiment. In the case of jelly, it requires about 65% by weight of sugar for this growth–inhibiting effect to be observed.

A third and final example of the growth inhibitors available to the food industry is propionic acid; it is a natural acid which gives the characteristic tart flavor to Swiss cheese. In bread, propionic acid prevents the growth of bread molds for a limited time. A variety of other acids are also useful in foods for the same reason. For example, sulfur dioxide (forming sulfuric acid) is used in fruits, and nitrite (forming nitric acid) is used in meats such as bologna, hams, hot dogs, and pastrami.

III. SANITATION

A. "CLEAN" VS. "SANITARY"

Many people think in terms of a "clean" environment when it comes to food, its preparation, and consumption. From biblical times this term has generally been interpreted to mean "sound and healthy" or "wholesome for consumption" in that clean food did not transmit disease. Early peoples had to rely on

TABLE 5
Rating of Selected Foods
Expressed as "Low" or "High"
in Acid Content[a]

Food	Acid rating
Low-acid foods	
Bananas	Low
Beans, green	Low
Beef	Low
Broccoli	Low
Chicken	Low
Corn	Low
Fish	Low
Lettuce	Low
Milk	Low
Spinach	Low
High-acid foods	
Apples	High
Buttermilk	High
Grapes	High
Grapefruit	High
Limes	High
Olives	High
Oranges	High
Plums	High
Tomatoes	High

[a] Where pH 4.6 is taken as the cutoff point according to the Food and Drug Administration criteria for acidity in foods.

their eyes to assess the cleanliness of food; therefore, the general understanding of cleanliness was simply that food was free of visible dirt and debris.

With the development of disciplines of zoology, microbiology, and others in more recent times, it was discovered that there are living organisms that cannot be seen with the naked eye. In the 19th century, Louis Pasteur of France demonstrated that microorganisms could lead to the spoilage of food. Eventually, this discovery led to the germ theory of disease which states that microbial diseases can be transmitted or "communicated" from one person to another through vectors including food, dishes, and utensils (Section I.B).

The discovery of pathogens and nonpathogens in and on foods added another, major dimension to the old concept of cleanliness. A new term had to be coined to encompass the additional information: "sanitary". Like the old term, "clean", this new one still refers to food that is wholesome for consumption, but its use symbolically recognizes the need to control disease–causing factors that are visible and invisible.

B. PERSONAL HYGIENE

The first thing to do when entering the kitchen is to wash your hands at the sink. Keep a bar of soap there along with a fresh hand towel. Take time to wash thoroughly. Be careful with your clean hands; anything they touch might contaminate them. During meal preparation, wash your hands after handling dirty dishes, touching the floor, and always after handling raw animal products and any equipment these products may have touched.

Many people believe that wearing clear plastic gloves helps to cut down on the transmission of microbes in the kitchen. If properly used, this is true. Some people, though, have the wrong perception about gloves, thinking that it is hands that cause food poisoning. They do not understand that the microbes on the foods do it. It does not matter whether or not you have on gloves; a gloved hand can still transmit disease. Unfortunately, gloves may only serve to give a false sense of security to users. It is not uncommon to see the gloved hand preparing meat one moment, then holding a telephone receiver, then picking something up off the floor, and so on.

Another major concern is the contamination of food with your own fecal microbes. This happens when you use the toilet, but do not wash your hands afterward. Fecal microbes can get on your hands during wiping; they are still there after you leave the bathroom. Everything you touch is inoculated with these pathogens. In the kitchen, they find a welcome environment in which to grow in the food you are preparing to eat. It is imperative that you wash your hands well after using the toilet, especially if you have diarrhea with a messy cleanup. Additionally, wash your hands after voiding; the genitals are in close proximity to the anus and cross contamination is possible.

C. FOOD SANITATION

Sanitary measures are those that break the chain of infection through which microbes are transmitted. The chain begins with the purchase of food at the grocery store. All food should be regarded as contaminated or potentially contaminated. What is done with this food after bringing it out of the store is critical to determining whether it will be a vector for disease. The objective is to handle food in ways that do not allow for the growth of pathogens or excess numbers of spoilage organisms which can also cause illness in PWAs.

1. Transport

After purchasing food, take it directly home. If stops are made on the way home, cold food can warm up and enter the temperature danger zone (Section II.D.2), activating pathogens and making the food unwholesome.

2. Storage

When arriving home from the grocery store, put the food away promptly beginning with refrigerated and frozen items. Cold foods should be stored cold.

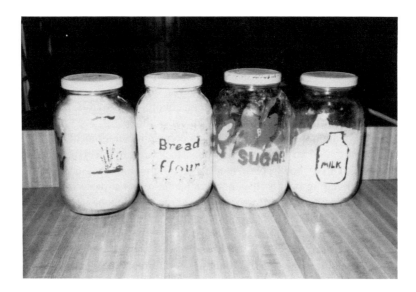

FIGURE 4. Dry foods are properly stored in glass or metal containers that are insect and rodent proof. Shown here in 1-gallon glass jars are (left to right) whole wheat flour, bread flour, sugar, and nonfat dry milk. Hand painted artwork on the jars gives them a friendly, personal touch that individualizes the kitchen.

Make sure your refrigerator keeps food below the temperature danger zone (Section II.D.2). Frozen foods should be kept rock solid; there should not be any thawing (indicated by soft spots) in the freezer. Arrange food in the freezer and refrigerator so that forced, cold/cool air can circulate well. Keep the appliance clean so that it does not become a vector for disease.

Foods stored at room temperature should be kept in glass jars or tin containers to prevent insect infestation (Figure 4). This is particularly important for flour. All products should be kept in a cabinet or closet that does not permit access by rodents because they are vectors for disease. Roaches and flies are difficult to exclude from the kitchen, but there are good roach control products on the market. Flies can be largely controlled by excluding them from your house; a screen door and screened windows provide good control. Additionally, the use of fly paper and traps can help.

Periodically, storage cabinets and drawers should be vacuumed to remove roach excretions and any other debris. Inspect cabinets for evidence of rodents, including droppings and points of access. Floors and cabinet surfaces should all be washed regularly. While many prefer the "organic" or "designer" look in a kitchen decor, white remains one of the best choices because dirt shows up readily. Simply look at the surfaces of the counter, appliances, and cabinets to know whether they are clean or not. The presence of dirt indicates the need for cleaning, not for a change of paint to a darker color.

3. Preparation

Food is often mishandled during its preparation in several ways. The most important way is to allow food being prepared to come into contact with other contaminated foods or contaminated kitchen equipment such as cutting boards, knives, utensils, counters, etc. A second way to mishandle frozen or cold food is to leave it out in the kitchen at room temperature. As it warms, the temperature moves into the danger zone, and pathogens thrive.

It is understood that each piece of food preparation equipment and kitchen countertops should be sanitary every time they are used. This rule includes countertops, knives, bowls, pans, utensils of various sorts, measuring cups and spoons, and cutting boards. It is not acceptable to use a piece of equipment during the preparation of different foods without washing the item in between uses. Failure to sanitize food preparation equipment and kitchen countertops in between contact with different foods is a major reason for cross contamination and foodborne illness.

In order to meet the need for sanitary food preparation equipment, you must first have items that are capable of being sanitized. Stainless steel is the material of choice for most applications such as utensils, pots, and pans and even for countertops, sinks, cabinet doors, and shelves. High–quality stainless steel is relatively expensive, but it is very durable. Alternatives to stainless steel include various plastics for countertops, utensils, and cutting boards. Porcelain is also popular for surfacing stoves, refrigerators, mixers, and other appliances.

One material that is not acceptable is wood, because it is a porous material. These pores trap microbes, protecting them from being dislodged and/or destroyed by soap and water or even sanitizing agents. It is not advisable to put wooden utensils (spoons, paddles, forks, etc.) or cutting boards in the dishwasher, because the heat could cause warping or splitting. Consequently, wooden equipment can be a ready vector for disease by transferring microbes from one food to the next (cross contamination) even if it has been washed in between uses. Only white plastic, dishwasher safe cutting boards should be used in your kitchen. They should be washed in the dishwasher routinely if not every day and always after contact with raw animal products. Give up wooden utensils; use stainless steel or dishwasher–safe plastic items.

In general, it is a good idea to separate meal preparation into two parts. The first part includes anything with raw animal products. The second part does not include raw animal products. Deal with raw animal parts first. After you have finished, clean the kitchen as described below and then proceed to the second part. Following this strategy with care will prevent the cross contamination of raw and cooked foods and foods made with and without raw animal products.

All raw animal products should be regarded as being contaminated with pathogens. Any surface these products touch becomes contaminated. Again, all equipment and countertops used during preparation should be sanitized. In addition, keep a mental list of everything touched in the kitchen during preparation such as handles on the stove or refrigerator, spice cans, salt box, and so on; all of these items must be washed, too, as they might be contaminated.

4. Food Processing to Control Microbes
a. *Ideal: Sterile Food*

Ideally, food for immunocompromised persons would be sterile, without any living microbes. When food handling techniques are adequate, the risk for foodborne illness and opportunistic infections decreases greatly. It is possible to process food to render it sterile. Conventional methods using dry heat or steam have the disadvantage of destroying sensory attributes such as color and texture. The perfect method for sterilizing food would not raise its temperature at all.

Modern food technology makes this possible through irradiation. This process makes use of a radioactive source of energy to send radiation into the food product. The radiation instantly kills microbes in and on the surface of food, but it does not raise its temperature.

Irradiation has not been embraced in the United States, perhaps because people are suspicious of food processed this way; some think the food might be radioactive after processing. There is no evidence to support this belief after nearly 50 years of testing.

Another reason why irradiation has not caught on is the cost; it is a very expensive process that cannot be performed in the home, a manufacturing facility being required. Hence, the perfect food technology for the immunocompromised consumer is not available, in the practical sense.

b. *Practical: Sanitary Food*

Fortunately, food does not have to be sterile to be wholesome. Conventional heating methods using a stove and/or oven will produce sanitary food without severe heat treatment. In most cases, food is cooked without great loss of desirable sensory attributes. Importantly, pathogens will be destroyed, but heat–loving, spoilage microbes can survive (Section II.D.3); low levels of spoilage organisms should not present a problem in the gut even for immunocompromised persons.

Food processors are familiar with food that is sanitary, yet contains live microbes. For example, canned foods are only heated to destroy pathogens, but spoilage–causing, heat–loving microbes remain alive inside the can. These products are considered to be "commercially sterile". Examples of commer-cially sterile products include pasteurized milk and most canned foods. Again, these foods could be sterilized through severe heat treatment, but sensory qualities would deteriorate.

All foods cannot be prepared to the standard of *commercial* sterility. Raw animal products should be cooked to the point of *total* sterility (no living microbes). Statistics indicate that these foods are very often the vectors of foodborne illness. This is a simple reflection of the nature of the environment in these foods (Section II): it is highly favorable to the growth of microbes, especially pathogens, because of the common exposure of animals to soil and fecal material (Section VI.A).

c. Microwaving

Microwaving is a method of cooking that became popular in the 1980s. It deserves special mention because some people expect food to behave the same way in a microwave oven as it does in a conventional oven, but the fact is that there are important differences. Sometimes the lack of understanding results in undercooked food because it is not processed in the unit correctly to allow for even heating to a high (hot) temperature. Unfortunately, this greatly increases the risk for food poisoning.

If you want to cook with a microwave oven, use a microwave–safe turntable to rotate the food during cooking. This will eliminate hot and cold spots to ensure even heating. The second item you need is a thermometer. Be sure it is a microwave–safe thermometer if you leave it in the food during operation of the unit. Test the temperature of food at the center portion. It should always read above the temperature danger zone (60°C or 140°F), but it is generally recommended that food temperatures approach the well–done stage (82°C or 180°F). Note that well–done food readily shows loss of sensory qualities.

Contrary to popular notions, microwaving does not cook food from the inside out. Food is penetrated to a depth of about 1 to 2 centimeters (about 1/2 inch) by the waves of radiation. The water molecules in this area of penetration get hot because of the energy bombardment. The heat produced marches into the interior of the food just the way it does in the conventional heat method.

Some people worry that the surface of microwaved foods does not get hot enough to kill pathogens. You do not have to worry about this because it is not true. The surface does get very hot, and microbes are killed. The reason that the surface does not seem to get hot is that the chamber of a microwave oven does not get hot during operation. Therefore, heat can radiate out of the food and into the oven chamber; this results in a cooling effect at the surface. By way of contrast, in a conventional oven, where the chamber is hot, heat cannot escape from the food into the oven because the chamber is already hot; instead, the presence of heat in the chamber tends to cause a buildup of heat in the food.

d. Washing

Besides heating, washing is a practical procedure for reducing the microbial content of food. Washing simply remove microbes. Food is thoroughly cleaned under running water. A scrub brush is helpful providing that it is sanitary. The way to ensure this is to use it with hot, soapy water, which loosens microbes, dirt, and debris from the food as well as the brush. The food can be rinsed well to remove traces of soap after washing. Remember that an unsanitary scrub brush can be a potent source of microbial contamination because it comes into contact with so many other foods through dirty dishes, cutting boards, countertops, and utensils. Steps must be taken not to inoculate (contaminate) the food you are washing with a soiled brush.

e. Special Mention: Bulk Food Production

One mistake of special mention is that of letting hot food prepared in bulk, with large volume, remain on the stove to cool before storing it in the refrigerator. This practice is often justified on the basis that put "strain" would be placed on the refrigerator to cool the food if it was placed in the unit hot. Actually, it is dangerous to leave food out at room temperature to cool. As it passes through the temperature danger zone, pathogens will start to grow. For example, *Clostridium perfringens* from the air will land on the food and quickly establish colonies. As previously discussed, it does not take long for the contamination to become huge (Section II.D.2). The proper way to handle this situation is to "pan out" bulk foods; in other words, spoon out the food into shallow pans or plastic containers and put them into the refrigerator. In shallow pans, food produced in bulk can rapidly cool down to safe temperatures.

6. Sanitize Everything after Use

a. Washing Dishes by Hand

The Centers for Disease Control[2] has indicated that good quality household detergents are acceptable for use in the home for persons infected with HIV. There are a few important points to remember when washing dishes by hand. First, wash and/or scrub dishes in hot water. Food residue, grease, and microbes are all more soluble in hot water than cold. Second, use a grease–cutting dish soap. Soap dislodges and suspends food residues including grease and microbes from dishes. Use dish soap liberally; a little soap is required to lift each little bit of food residue. An excess will provide enough "power" to lift all the food residue. On the other hand, being overly conservative will leave some food residues on the dishes and incease the risk of foodborne illness. The third point is to rinse items well in hot water to carry away the dislodged food residue from the surface of dishes.

b. Sanitizing with Bleach

If you are having trouble with food poisoning at home, do not have hot water for washing and rinsing dishes, or want an added measure of safety, then it is a good idea to sanitize washed and rinsed dishes. A convenient and inexpensive method is to soak them in a solution made up from a sanitizing agent such as household bleach (Figure 5). Simply fill the up sink or a dishpan with water at about room temperature. Then add 3/4 cup bleach per gallon of water. Stir to mix. Immerse dishes, utensils, dishcloths, and other items for about 5 minutes. Remove and rinse; allow to air dry. Rinsing is especially important for items made of stainless steel because bleach is highly corrosive to that metal.

It is a good idea to wear heavy dish gloves when handling bleach and throughout the sanitizing process to protect your skin from the chemical effects

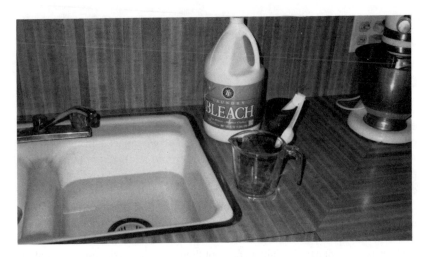

FIGURE 5.   Household bleach is an inexpensive, common sanitizing agent that is convenient to use. A soaking solution for dishes is made by adding 3/4 cup bleach for each gallon of water in the sink; immerse dishes for 5 minutes. *(True Value Brand Laundry Bleach, Fleming Companies, Inc.; Oklahoma City, OK)*

of bleach. Additionally, bleach will affect the colors of certain fabrics, especially blue jeans. You can protect your clothing by wearing an apron made of a synthetic blend or plastic.

If you find that the recommended bleach solution is too strong or too weak, then consider the range of effective concentrations suggested by the Centers for Disease Control:[2] 1 part bleach to 10 parts water (strong) all the way down to 1 part bleach to 100 parts water; weaker solutions require more time to be effective. Wear gloves for strong solutions.

A nice added benefit of using bleach is that it whitens and kills odors. Regular use will keep dishcloths looking clean and odor free. The same goes for dish brushes and scrubbers.

Not only does the bleach solution sanitize, but also it deodorizes and removes stains for general kitchen use (cabinet surfaces, floors, countertops, appliances). Additionally, it can be used in a sickroom to sanitize the bed, floor, furniture, and items (such as food trays, bed pans, pans or bowls to catch vomit, and rubber sheets) used by the person who is sick. Remember to wear gloves for your protection against the bleach solution, soiled dishes, and other sickroom equipment/items.

Caution: concentrated bleach from a jug is poisonous. You must store bleach in a location dedicated for kitchen chemicals. Examples of other kitchen chemicals include floor wax, window cleaner, silver polish, pine cleaner, and powdered scrubbing cleanser. Additionally, bleach is a strong chemical that should be handled with care. Wear gloves and eye covering when handling the jug; a fluid in a jug can shoot out of the top if it is set down with too much force.

c. *Automated Dishwashing*

Another way to sanitize dishes is with a dishwasher. These appliances are desirable for immunocompromised persons because of the high temperature wash and rinse cycles. The water temperatures reached inside the dishwasher are "hot hot". The dishwasher can stand a higher heat than a person can when doing dishes by hand because water that hot would burn. Another plus for dishwashers is the final sanitizing cycle using dry heat. Although it is an expensive method to sanitize dishes, it is convenient and very effective. Immunocompromised persons may wish to consider getting one; it greatly improves sanitation in the kitchen. Because the home is the second leading place of outbreaks of foodborne illness, purchasing a dishwasher should be seriously considered as one of the measures taken to assure kitchen sanitation. Purchase one with a sanitizing cycle (final heat drying).

7. Garbage

Often overlooked, a good system for handling garbage is necessary. Garbage is one of life's unpleasant realities to be dealt with. If left unchecked, garbage will smell and draw roaches, flies, other insects, and even rodents into your kitchen. The typical approach is to have a small plastic trash can in the kitchen lined with a bag. As the bag fills up, it is emptied into a large, main holding container or can outside the house. If the kitchen can is too large, the time interval between emptying will be too long and cause the problems listed above.

The outside disposal container can be metal or plastic; however, rodents generally seem to gnaw through plastic, but not metal. Line the can, keep the lid on tight, and make sure the surrounding area is kept clean. The presence of any food debris will attract dogs, cats, rodents and other wild animals such as raccoons and opossums. Do not come into contact with the fecal material of these animals; by taking great care to develop your own garbage disposal system, these animals will not visit.

Some people like to keep their main holding container in their garage (Figure 6). In this way, cans are protected from animals and the floor conditions can be strictly controlled. Odors can be contained by regular disposal of garbage on trash pickup days and by keeping the lid on tight. Garage storage also has the advantage of easy transfer of garbage from the kitchen to the main holding container. When the main container is outside, there is a tendency to wait on emptying the small kitchen cans until it is overflowing; that is too late. When the main container is in the next room, then "taking out the trash" is no chore at all.

IV. COMMON FOODBORNE INFECTIONS

There are many different microbes that may cause foodborne illness. Of these, a few have gained notoriety as important or emerging pathogens.

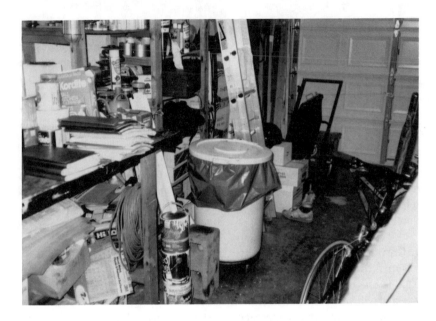

FIGURE 6. The large trash can for collecting kitchen and general household refuse can be located in the garage instead of outside; this placement makes it easier to keep small indoor trash cans emptied, resulting in a more sanitary home *(Rubbermaid Inc.; Wooster, OH)*

A. NOMENCLATURE

All microbes are classified into a "genus" or group, and that term is underlined or italicized. For example, *Salmonella* is the name of a group of pathogens typically found on poultry products. All of the members of the *Salmonella* genus are pathogens; thus it is acceptable to refer only to the genus. However, there are groups with some subgroups that cause disease, while others do not. In this case, it is necessary to refer to both the genus and species or subgroup of the microbe. For example, *Vibrio parahaemolyticus* is an example of one particular intestinal microbe causing foodborne disease in man.

B. INFECTIONS AND INTOXICATIONS

Foodborne illness comes in two types: infections and intoxications. Infections result when living cells are ingested and illness results; intake of dead (cooked) cells does not result in illness. Intoxications result from eating food containing poison produced by microbes; in this case, living organisms do not have to be consumed to cause illness. The focus of interest here is mostly on foodborne infections because they can lead to opportunistic infections (Section I.C).

C. SYMPTOMS

Symptoms of foodborne illness can be specific to a microbe or generalized across many different types of microbes. Of the five microbes discussed

TABLE 6
General Information on *Salmonella*, the Leading Cause
of Foodborne Illness in the United States

Importance
  The major cause of reported outbreaks and cases of foodborne illness; persons
  with AIDS are 20 times more susceptible to infection than are healthy individuals
Disease vector
  Raw animal products
Uniqueness
  All poultry should be assumed to be contaminated; handle with caution
Type of illness
  Infection
Mechanism by which illness is caused
  Must ingest viable cells which produce an enterotoxin in the intestine
Onset of symptoms
  12 to 24 hours
Clinical manifestations
  Gastroenteritis including fever, diarrhea, abdominal cramps, pain in abdomen,
  vomiting, pseudoappendicitis, and nausea

in this section that cause intestinal infections, all result in the same general complaint of "classic gastroenteritis". Symptoms include nausea, vomiting, abdominal cramps, diarrhea, chills, and fever. The degree of sickness, from mild to intense, is dependent on the number and virulence or poison potential of living cells consumed in the contaminated food. In healthy persons, a vigorous immune response may contain the illness quickly, within 1 or 2 days. By contrast, you may experience symptoms for a week or much longer.

One microbe, *Staphylococcus aureus*, discussed in this section, causes an intoxication. It is not a likely source of infection through the gut. *Staphylococcus aureus* is discussed because it normally resides in the nasal passages, and this makes it readily available to contaminate cuts or sores on your hands or body. For example, wiping the nose with a hand contaminates the surface of the hand; moreover, if there is an open cut or sore, then it can get infected. If it goes unchecked because of an immunocompromised condition, then a whole–body, opportunistic infection may result (Section I.C).

D. *Salmonella*

Long considered to be the number 1 source of food poisoning in the United States, *Salmonella* now takes a back seat to *Campylobacter* (Table 6). All species of the former genus are pathogens, and some are quite virulent. It is an intestinal microbe found in the fecal excretions of many animals; living organisms are excreted. Flies, roaches, and rodents coming into contact with feces pick up *Salmonella* where it is present and transfer it to your food, drink, and kitchen equipment and surfaces. Avoid this contamination by controlling the access of flies, roaches, and rodents to the home.

Salmonella is notorious for being present on the skin, feathers, and feet of poultry. The reason for this is that birds are indiscriminant about their bowel movements. They will walk in their own excreta as well as eat feed that has been coated with it. Consequently, the surface of their bodies is contaminated, and they continually reinfect themselves with the microbe by eating it. During the kill process, *Salmonella* is unavoidably spread everywhere on the chicken carcass, but the levels are low when properly handled. It is up to the consumer to carefully protect the poultry purchase in order that the levels do not increase to an unsafe level.

The following description of an outbreak is provided by the Centers for Disease Control:[3]

Outbreak of *Salmonella enteritidis* Infection
Associated with Consumption of Raw Shell Eggs, 1991
(Paraphrased)

During October 1991, 15 persons who ate at a restaurant during a 9-day period developed gastroenteritis. Symptoms of illness included diarrhea, vomiting, fever, abdominal cramping, nausea, and chills. Of 13 patrons seeking medical care, 6 had to be hospitalized. Of the 15 ill patrons, 14 had eaten Caesar salad; none of 11 other well patrons had eaten Caesar salad. Caesar salad was implicated as the disease vector.

The Caesar salad dressing was prepared early in the morning by combining 36 yolks from hand–cracked eggs with olive oil, anchovies, garlic, and warm water. Neither lemon juice nor vinegar was included in the recipe. Batches of Caesar dressing were prepared daily….The dressing was refrigerated until the restaurant opened, when it was placed in a chilled compartment in the salad preparation area for approximately 8 to 12 hours until the restaurant closed. By the time a restaurant inspection was conducted, the restaurant had eliminated Caesar salad from the menu. However, at the time of the inspection, the temperature of other salad dressings present in this compartment was 15.6°C (60°F), in the danger zone.

The vector of this outbreak was the egg. Although clean, its surface was undoubtedly contaminated with *Salmonella*. When the eggs were cracked, organisms most likely got onto the hands of the food service worker. As he separated the yolks from the whites, the yolks became contaminated as they touched his hands. Then the microbes "waited" until the temperature was favorable for growth. Note that the addition of lemon juice or vinegar might have prevented the growth of *Salmonella* by increasing the acidity of the salad dressing (Section II.F).

E. *Campylobacter jejuni*
This microbe has become important in the last 10 years, although it has been a source of food poisoning since long before then (Table 7). Food

TABLE 7
General Information on *Campylobacter*, an Emerging Pathogen

Importance
> Statistics from the Centers for Disease Control indicate that campylobecteriosis is not as important as salmonellosis even though both are found in the intestinal tracts of the same land animals; improved methods of detection and identification may increase the number of outbreaks attributable to this microbe

Disease vector
> Raw animal products

Uniqueness
> Easily destroyed by heat and inactivated by cold (refrigerator temperatures)

Type of illness
> Infection

Mechanism by which illness is caused
> Must ingest viable cells; once inside, cells produce a toxin (enterotoxin) leading to gastroenteritis

Onset of symptoms
> Several days to a week (makes it difficult to trace vector)

Clinical manifestations
> Classic gastroenteritis including fever, diarrhea, abdominal cramps, and pain in abdomen

microbiologists were not able to easily screen and identify *Campylobacter jejuni* until the early 1980s. The microbe is thought to be a frequent contaminant of raw animal products because it is normally resides in the intestinal tract of animals.

The following description of an outbreak is provided by the Centers for Disease Control:[4]

Campylobacter Outbreak Associated with
Certified Raw Milk Products—California

On May 31, 1984, 28 kindergarten children and seven adults from a private school of 240 students in Whittier, California, visited a certified raw milk bottling plant in southern California, where they were given ice cream, kefir, and certified raw milk. Three to six days later, several of the group began to experience fever and gastroenteritis. Ultimately, nine children and three adults became ill, and most of them were absent from school. Studies on stools from these 12 individuals for routine bacterial pathogens showed nine positive and three negative for *Campylobacter jejuni*. Stools were obtained from nine non–ill children in another kindergarten class; these stools did not yield *C. jejuni*. The only common foods these children (ill and non–ill) ate were hamburgers, which are provided every Thursday to their school by a fast–food hamburger chain. No one else in the school became sick.

TABLE 8
General Information on *Staphylococcus aureus*, a Leading Cause of Foodborne Illness

Importance
Common microbe producing foodborne illness by intoxication

Disease vector
Combination dishes with meat which have been held within the temperature danger zone

Uniqueness
Organisms usually come from nose of man; a food handler can infect himself by wiping his nose on his hand; the resultant infection on the hand can turn into an opportunistic infection in an immunocompromised person

Type of illness
Intoxication by food; infection by transmission to cuts or sores on the hands

Mechanism by which illness is caused
Toxin if contaminated food eaten; viable cells cause infection in cuts and sores

Onset of symptoms
Rapid onset (about 4 hours) to toxin because viable cells are not needed to produce the toxin inside the gut; an infection through a cut or sore can rapidly progress (days) in the immunocompromised individual

Clinical manifestations
Intoxication produces classic gastroenteritis: fever, diarrhea, abdominal cramps, and pain in abdomen

It was concluded that the raw milk product(s) served as a vector for the transmission of *C. jejuni*, leading to disease in some individuals. Many factors could have accounted for the fact that not all visiting children and staff got ill; however, one of the most likely factors is the volume of contaminated raw milk consumed.

F. *Staphylococcus aureus*

Staphylococcus aureus does not have to produce an infection in man to cause illness (Table 8). Disease is caused by a toxin produced by the microbes working in food before it is eaten. The toxin may challenge the body's immune system, but it cannot become an opportunistic infection with the potential to kill. Ordinarily, this type of food poisoning, by toxin, is not deadly.

It is probably more important to consider that *Staphylococcus aureus* organisms are typically living in the nose of man. A very common problem is for persons with cuts or sores on their hands to wipe their noses with those same hands. This transfers organisms from the nose to the cut, and infection gets underway in the cut. This rightfully can be termed an opportunistic infection because it will proceed to a greater extent with a weakened immune system.

G. *Clostridium perfringens*

The notable thing about *Clostridium perfringens* is that it is a spore–forming microbe (Table 9). When conditions are harsh, it has the ability to transform

TABLE 9
General Information on *Clostridium perfringens*, a Leading Cause of Foodborne Illness in the United States

Importance
Very common cause of foodborne illness

Disease vector
Combination dishes, especially ones with meat

Uniqueness
Clostridia are present in air and dust as spores; they are always present and pose a ready danger for foods held in the temperature danger zone

Type of illness
Infection

Mechanism by which illness is caused
Innoculated food must be held at warm temperature, but below 60°C; clostridia are mesophiles; large numbers of cells must be ingested to cause illness; inside gut, spores are released and spore coats irritate gut lining, leading to enteritis

Onset of symptoms
8 to 12 hours

Clinical manifestations
Classic gastroenteritis: fever, diarrhea, abdominal cramps, and pain in abdomen

TABLE 10
General Information on *Vibrio parahaemolyticus*, an Emerging Pathogen Found in Seafood Products

Importance
An emerging pathogen for seafood

Disease vector
Intestinal tract of seafood products

Uniqueness
This microbe can withstand the salty ocean; its counterparts, *Salmonella* and *Campylobacter,* cannot tolerate the salt of the oceans

Type of illness
Infection, virulent

Mechanism by which illness is caused
Not well known; the microbe probably produces an enterotoxin or somehow irritates the gut lining

Onset of symptoms
12 to 24 hours

Clinical manifestations
Classic gastroenteritis: fever, diarrhea, abdominal cramps, and pain in abdomen

its outer wall into a very tough envelope; it waits inside until the environmental conditions are favorable again. Spores are highly mobile, being able to move in the air with dust. They are everywhere around us. This is an important reason not to leave food on the stove uncovered to cool. Spores can land on it and become active.

TABLE 11
General Information on *Listeria monocytogenes*, an Emerging Cause of Foodborne Illness

Importance
   Persons with AIDS are 200 to 300 times more likely to contract listeriosis than
   are healthy persons

Disease vector
   Products made from unpasteurized milk, especially soft cheeses

Uniqueness
   Grows in the refrigerator and in the presence of salt; therefore, it is well
   positioned to grow on cheese, a salted product stored in the refrigerator

Type of illness
   Meningitis; whole body infection (opportunistic infection)

Mechanism by which illness is caused
   Infection of the body; infection of the gut

Onset of symptoms
   8 to 12 hours

Clinical manifestations
   Classic gastroenteritis: fever, diarrhea, abdominal cramps, and pain in abdomen

H. *Vibrio parahaemolyticus*

Vibrio is similar to *Salmonella* in that both organisms are found in the intestinal tracts of animals (Table 10). However, *Vibrio* is found in animals that inhabit the oceans and is salt tolerant; *Salmonella* is not salt tolerant. In fact, salt is a growth inhibitor for many microbes (Section II.G). *Vibrio* is said to be an emerging pathogen because the number of reported cases of food poisoning has increased sharply in recent years.

I. *Listeria monocytogenes*

Listeria monocytogenes has been associated with disease in soft cheeses made from unpasteurized (raw) milk (Table 11). Implicated kinds include Mexican–style "white" cheese, feta, Brie, Camembert, and blue–veined cheeses. There is no evidence to suggest that hard types of cheeses such as cheddar, yogurt, cottage cheese, or cream cheese should be avoided.

Some individuals encourage eating products made from raw milk because of alleged health benefits of raw milk; however, the purpose of pasteurization is to kill microbes that would cause foodborne disease and possibly even opportunistic infections in the body.

Immunocompromised individuals are 200 to 300 times more likely to contract listeriosis than healthy individuals. Illness will be of a longer duration than for healthy persons because of the weakened immune system, and the chances of it progressing from the gut into the body through the bloodstream are higher, too. At the stage of whole–body involvement, the patient would be facing a life–threatening, opportunistic infection. This level of risk just to drink raw milk is unacceptable.

V. EATING IN: HOME

A. RAW ANIMAL PRODUCTS

Raw animal products are a frequent vector of disease. The reason for this problem is twofold. First, these raw foods provide microbes with favorable living environments (Section II). Second, animals are exposed to pathogens in the normal course of their existence. They are generally indiscrete in bowel activity and come in contact with feces; and they have close contact with soil, which harbors many types of microorganisms including pathogens.

1. Eggs

Before eating egg dishes, make sure that there are no raw or partially cooked egg products in them. Do not eat hollandaise or salad dressings that may contain raw eggs. Egg products should be cooked to the well done or hard–cooked stage; do not be afraid to refuse undercooked food. Fried eggs should be cooked on both sides; the yolk should be hard. Scrambled eggs should be firm, not runny. Be suspicious of egg custard products such as pies and ice cream. Eat only those custard products that have been commercially prepared; do not eat those that are homemade because the controls on production are not strict enough to ensure a reasonable degree of safety.

2. Meat of Land Animals

Meat should be firm to the touch when hard cooked; undercooked meat will deform at the center under the pressure of a fork or finger. Another quick test is to cut open the meat to see whether it is "bloody" (cut by the bone for poultry). While red–colored juice is not actually blood (animals are bled after slaughter), its presence does indicate that the meat has not been cooked to the well–done stage since large amounts of juice are lost at that cooking end point. According to these criteria, steak tartar (raw or bloody steak) also is off the list of recommended foods to eat.

3. Seafood

The consumption of raw seafood, as in raw oysters or raw fish (sushi), is dangerous for someone who is immunocompromised. It should be obvious that any raw food may contain high levels of pathogens. When fish is gutted, intestinal organisms (*Vibrio parahaemolyticus*) may contaminate the flesh. Only cooking will destroy these pathogens. Boiled seafood presents another problem. Shrimp and scallops become rubbery when overcooked, and may be undercooked in order to prevent this undesirable texture change. Unfortunately, pathogens may escape destruction. Shrimp are a problem because the intestinal tract cannot be easily removed, and even if it were, the flesh would be contaminated. Shrimp must be well cooked or there will be a risk for foodborne illness from *Vibrio*.

B. RAW FRUITS AND VEGETABLES

Whether a person is healthy or infected with HIV, everyone should always clean raw fruits and vegetables. Typically, the surfaces are contaminated with low levels of pathogens and spoilage microbes tht come either from the soil in which the products were grown or the wash water used to clean products after harvesting.

Ordinarily, cleaning in the home is limited to rinsing in tap water. This treatment does remove visible dirt and debris, some of the microbes, and possibly chemical residues present on the surface. Healthy persons can easily tolerate the typically low level of remaining microbial contamination, but PWAs may find that even low levels are problematic because of their weakened immune status (Section I.C). More detailed instructions for washing are given elsewhere (Section III.C.4.d).

C. BREAD

Bread is stable microbiologically due to its low water content and low water activity level (Sections II.A and II.B). It will keep well on the counter or shelf for several days, especially if it contains preservatives such as propionic acid, butylated hydroxyanisole (BHA), or butylated hydroxytoluene (BHT). After a while, mold will begin to grow despite the presence of any preservatives. When evidence of mold (usually black or blue "dust" on the surface) can be seen, then the entire loaf should be thrown out.

When color is present on the surface, the microbe has successfully tunneled throughout the loaf. In other words, the mold has established a network of tubes inside the crumb of the bread (white part); then it "congratulates itself" by sending flags to the surface for everyone to see. Do not try to cut away the mold; this does not work because the mold has already penetrated way beneath the surface. Throw the loaf away. Besides the question of ingesting live cells of mold, these microbes are now recognized to produce toxins that can be harmful to humans. Do not eat moldy bread.

Learn to recognize how long bread can be kept before it molds. If a whole loaf cannot be eaten before that time period, then freeze the bread in the plastic bag. Bread freezes wonderfully. Simply toast it right out of the freezer, or let it thaw on your sanitary cutting board if toast is not desired.

D. PASTEURIZED DAIRY PRODUCTS

Cheese is like bread in that mold is undesirable, unless that is how the cheese is traditionally processed (for example, blue cheese). Green or blue mold spots, usually circular, on the surface of old cheese mean it is time to throw it out. Remember that mold in cheese works the same way as it does in bread. When it can be seen on the surface, it has already invaded the interior. Do not try to cut away the mold, because it is not possible to see the extensive network of tunnels. Again, molds produce toxins that are unhealthy for you to eat.

Milk should always be pasteurized. Never drink raw milk. Be very careful never to handle raw food, especially raw animal products, when also handling a jug of milk. Milk is an excellent growth medium for pathogens including *Campylobacter* and *Salmonella*.

E. COMMERCIALLY PACKAGED PRODUCTS

Many commercially packaged foods display a "sell by" date on the package. Look for this date before purchasing any item. There should be enough days remaining to allow consumption of all of the product by the "sell by" date. It is a common practice for shoppers to stock up on foods when at the grocery store, but the result may be that the extra foods "expire", and spoilage organisms begin to grow inside. With a weakened immune status, large numbers of nonpathogenic microbes in unopened packages can still cause illness.

VI. EATING OUT: RESTAURANTS

A. THE PROBLEM WITH FOOD SERVICE EMPLOYEES

There are two places where food poisoning outbreaks occur with great frequency: the home and food service facilities, including cafeterias, delicatessens, and restaurants. Of these, restaurants were consistently responsible for more outbreaks over the time period from 1983 to 1987.[5] Therefore, one must be much more careful when dining out than when eating at home.

As a consumer in a restaurant paying for food to be prepared and served, a patron has a reasonable expectation that sanitary measures will be followed. Common experience, though, has shown again and again that one should always be cautious when someone else is preparing the food. Despite strict government standards for the construction, equipage, and operation of restaurants as well as periodic inspections by the local health department, outbreaks of foodborne illness cannot be stopped.

There are two important reasons for outbreaks. First, food is a natural vector for disease (Section I.B). Second, it is very easy to mishandle food. This second point is made clear by data from the Centers for Disease Control showing that the leading cause of food poisoning is improper storage or holding temperatures, and the second most frequent cause is poor personal hygiene of the food handler.

A chronic problem with restaurants seems to be with unknowledgeable and inexperienced employees. Apparently they fail to follow the basic rules of sanitary food handling and service that would be used at home or that commercial food processors use in their manufacturing plants. It is generally agreed that education and training of restaurant employees are two solutions to the problem.

Unfortunately, it is difficult to educate and train restaurant employees because they tend to be a mobile work force. Turnover is great because wages are at the minimum level, and the work is low in status. Furthermore, some employees do not plan to make their restaurant job a long–term position. They view it as temporary work until something better comes along; consequently, there may be little or no commitment to doing well. Management also shares in the blame because it may not invest the required time, energy, and money in recruiting, training, and retaining good employees.

B. AVOIDING ILLNESS
1. Patronize by Reputation
Almost all restaurants are cited at inspection time for a few minor violations because they are complex operations where many things can go wrong. Some, though, tend to have more trouble than others, and these few may be repeat offenders. Common problems indicating poor sanitation in the kitchen are rodent and roach infestation and slime (microbial contamination) in the ice machine. Significant problems in food handling include steam table and walk–in refrigerator operation at unsafe temperatures and unacceptably high risk for cross contamination of food in the kitchen, sometimes due to the lack of dedicated preparation areas for different types of foods.

Seek out and patronize only restaurants with good reputations. Good food service operations will receive high marks at inspection time year after year. Their success is no accident; it can always be attributed to a knowledgeable and experienced staff who goes out of its way to maintain a sanitary kitchen and follow proper food handling procedures. The zeal of these establishments comes from their desire to build and maintain a loyal clientele—a major food poisoning outbreak would be a public relations disaster.

One way to sort out the good restaurants from the bad is to look for newspaper reports, local magazine surveys, or even "restaurant reports" by local news shows. It is a good idea to be sure that the report or survey is independent of the businesses being reviewed; this requirement is necessary to obtain the most objective information.

2. Order "Safe" Foods
Eat at restaurants that serve relatively safe food — food that is hard to abuse. Pizza is an excellent example. Bread, pizza sauce, and cheese are all naturally preserved. Meat (beef, chicken, fish, pork) are good bets, too, especially if you can order them freshly cooked to the well–done stage. Stay away from meats that have been precooked because you cannot be certain they have been held out of the danger zone. Do not eat food that has been kept "piping hot" under a heat lamp. Heat lamps do not keep food out of the temperature danger zone. Do not eat any combination dish containing meat such as spaghetti sauce or sloppy joe. These dishes can be held in the steam table for hours; the required monitoring of temperature to keep them truly hot may be lacking. See comments about eggs and seafood in Sections V.A.1 and V.A.3.

3. Facilities Supervised by Dietitians

An important assurance of safety in a food service facility is the presence of a dietitian. This health care professional has extensive formal college training in the safe operation of food service facilities. There are many functions of the dietitian in a food service facility. One function of great importance is the checking of food temperatures to be sure that cold foods are cold and hot foods are hot. It is not uncommon to see a dietitian inserting a thermometer into a food pan on the steam table and adjusting the temperature of the heating element as necessary.

The food service business manager tends to perceive of food as a vehicle for making money. By contrast, the dietitian thinks of food as nourishment. This difference in perceptions makes a critical difference in attitudes and priorities in the facility. The dietitian is likely to focus on quality food service while the business manager might be willing to overlook some elements of quality in order to achieve maximum dollar return.

Generally speaking, cafeterias in schools and health care facilities are supervised by dietitians. For example, the cafeterias found in hospitals, nursing homes, schools, and colleges might be run by dietitians. Many of these are open to the public. They are good places to eat for persons with compromised immune systems.

VII. FOREIGN TRAVEL

The basic rules for travel are to drink bottled water or juices only. Wipe off the bottle cap before opening. Sometimes juice comes in a paper "brick" pack (looks like a brick), but this may be too much to drink — throw away the leftover. If bottled water or juices are not available, then boil your own water in a sanitary pan. If you desire ice, then make it yourself from boiled water because freezing does not kill microbes. While the consumption of alcoholic beverages may not be desirable (Chapter 7), it is worth mentioning that beer and wine are preserved, safe forms of water and grape juice, respectively. If you must have something to drink and nothing else is available, then beer and wine may hold you until something else can be obtained.

Restaurants with an American flavor may be disappointing when visiting a foreign country. It is only natural to want to try a little of the local cuisine. It can be done if you are careful. The first rule is to eat in upscale restaurants where cooked food is served very hot. Look at the fare displayed on the menu and check out the clientele. These two indicators will tell a lot. Safe bets include pancakes and waffles; they are a wonderful and different experience in European countries. Some popular restaurants will offer spicy foods with bread. This should be safe because many spices retard the growth of microbes. There is just no substitute for the French bread–and–cheese meal; it is nourishing and delicious. Try to determine whether the cheese is made from pasteurized milk; customs vary outside of the United States. Hard cheese is a safer bet than soft varieties because it contains less water to support microbes.

Fruits and vegetables present a difficult problem for the traveler. As a general rule, do not eat anything that you cannot peel yourself; this means avoiding salads. By contrast, bread is almost always safe, as well as hard, dry, and spicy sausage in which you can taste the preservative nitrite. Beef and pork sausage will have an intense pink color inside due to the presence of nitrite; look for the color. Peel off the outer casing of the sausage before eating it.

Last, do not eat any food served by street vendors. No matter what food it is, you simply cannot have reasonable confidence about its safety. It is the collective experience of travelers that foods from the street vendor are high risks for foodborne illnesses.

REFERENCES

1. **Keeton, W. T.,** *Biological Science*, 2nd ed., Norton, New York, 1972, chap. 21.
2. Centers for Disease Control, Summary: recommendations for preventing transmission of infection with human T–lymphotrophic virus type III/lymphadenopathy–associated virus in the workplace, *Morbidity Mortality Wkly. Rep.*, November 15, 34(45), 681, 1985.
3. Centers for Disease Control, Outbreak of *Salmonella enteritidis* infection associated with consumption of raw shell eggs, *Morbidity Mortality Wkly. Rep.*, May 29, 41(21), 369, 1992.
4. Centers for Disease Control, *Campylobacter* outbreak associated with certified raw milk products — California, *Morbidity Mortality Wkly. Rep.*, October 5, 1984, 33(39), 562, 1984.
5. **Bean, N. H., Griffin, P. M., Goulding, J. S., and Ivey, C. B.,** Foodborne disease outbreaks, 5–yr summary, 1983–1987, *Morbidity Mortality Wkly. Rep.*, 39(SS–1), 15, 1990.
6. *Composition of Foods*, Nos. 8–1 through 8–16, Agricultural Research Service, U.S. Department of Agriculture, Washington, D.C., 1976–1986.
7. **Banwart, G. J.,** *Basic Food Microbiology*, 2nd ed., Van Nostrand Reinhold, New York, 1989, chap. 4–6.
8. **Troller, J. A.,** Influence of water activity on microorganisms in foods, *Food Technol.*, 46(5), 76, 1980.
9. Centers for Disease Control, Listeriosis outbreak associated with Mexican–style cheese— California, *Morbidity Mortality Wkly. Rep.*, June 21, 34(24), 357, 1985.
10. Centers for Disease Control, Update: *Salmonella enteritidis* infections and shell eggs — United States, 1990, *Morbidity Mortality Wkly. Rep.*, December 21, 39(50), 909, 1990.
11. Centers for Disease Control, Update: foodborne listeriosis — United States, 1988–1990, *Morbidity Mortality Wkly. Rep.*, April 17, 41(15), 251, 1992.
12. **Frazier, W. C. and Westhoff, D. C.,** *Food Microbiology*, 4th ed., McGraw–Hill, New York, 1988.
13. **Liston, J.,** Microbial hazards of seafood consumption, *Food Technol.*, 44(12), 56, 1990.
14. **Martin, L. S., BcDougal, S., and Loskoski, S. L.,** Disinfection and inactivation of the human T lymphotropic virus type III/lymphadenopathy–associated virus, *J. Infect. Dis.*, 152, 400, 1985.

Chapter 7

ALCOHOL

J. F. Hickson, Jr.

CONTENTS

I. INTRODUCTION

A. LONG–RUN APPROACH TO HEALTH

Traditionally, nutritionists have been concerned with the drinking of alcoholic beverages by healthy persons because of the calories they contribute to the diet. Each gram of alcohol in these beverages contains 7 kcal of food energy. If added on top of the calories from foods eaten in a regular diet, then a positive energy balance (Chapter 1, Section V.A.2) can result leading to weight gain, possibly even a "beer belly".

A second concern for healthy persons is the relationship between alcohol consumption and the risk for chronic diseases. There does not appear to be any strong scientific data demonstrating that moderate drinking is a problem. Heavy or excess drinking, however, is well known to be associated with an increased risk for cirrhosis of the liver, elevated blood lipids and sugar, increased blood pressure and hemorrhagic stroke, and oropharyngeal, laryngeal, esophageal, liver, and breast cancers. It is important to note that the development of chronic diseases requires many years of heavy or excessive alcohol use.

B. SHORT–RUN APPROACH TO HEALTH

In contrast to well persons, immunocompromised persons need to take a short–run approach to successfully manage their health. There is comparatively little need to worry about becoming overweight or developing chronic diseases. Instead, they need to be on guard against those effects of alcohol consumption that might further weaken the immune system or continue the spread of HIV to susceptible tissues throughout the body.

C. THE HEALTH RISK OF ALCOHOL INTAKE

Two hypotheses have been put forward to define the health risks posed by alcohol consumption in the asymptomatic person living with HIV. Each of these centers around a different, basic assumption, but both hypotheses show great similarity to the models proposed to explain the potential for food additives to cause cancer in laboratory animals or humans.

The "threshold" hypothesis is traditional in its orientation. Accordingly, there is an acceptable range of alcohol intakes from zero up to some "safe" level of intake that is known as the "threshold". In Figure 1, the hypothetical level of safe intake is shown by the solid, vertical line.

When consumption exceeds the safe threshold of intake, then the hypothesis predicts that the risk of negative health consequences rapidly escalates. This is shown in Figure 1 by the dashed line which plots at an incline, beginning at the base of the threshold (solid vertical line). The maximum safe level of intake has not yet been defined, but it might correspond to the moderate drinking suggestion proposed in the 1990 "Dietary Guidelines".[1] The implication of this hypothesis is that you might be able to continue to enjoy your favorite cocktail

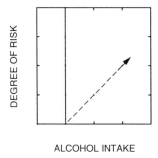

FIGURE 1.   The threshold hypothesis to explain the overall health risk of alcohol consumption states that there is a zone where limited intake is "safe" (i.e., without risk); however, when intake (dashed line) exceeds the threshold (solid line), then risk becomes proportional to intake.

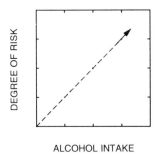

FIGURE 2.   The "zero–tolerance" hypothesis to explain the overall health risk of alcohol consumption states that there is no "safe" level of intake—all levels are met with some degree of risk, which increases in direct proportion to intake.

despite HIV infection (i.e., light or moderate alcohol consumption) providing that your doctor has not indicated otherwise.

The "zero–tolerance" hypothesis states that there is a risk to your health at any level of alcohol consumption (Figure 2). In other words, no level of alcohol intake is completely safe. Furthermore, as intake increases, so does the degree of risk. This is shown in Figure 2 as the dashed line proceeds on an incline in a direct, linear fashion to intake (Figure 2). Stated another way, the risk is directly proportional to the amount of alcohol consumed. For example, a small intake gives a small risk while a large intake gives a greater risk.

The interpretation of the zero tolerance model is traditional, dating back to the 1950s. In 1958, the U.S. Congress passed the Food Additives Amendment which contained the Delaney clause, also known as the zero tolerance provision. Accordingly, no cancer–causing food additives may be used in the food system of the United States because it is assumed that the risk of contracting cancer is directly proportional to the amount of exposure. Congress decided that no level of risk of cancer was acceptable for the American people.

If you apply the zero tolerance approach to HIV–positive persons, then you see that they do not have any room to maneuver in regard to alcohol consumption. Drinking alcohol might bring on the more rapid decline of the immune system along with AIDS and ultimately death (Chapter 1, Section III.B). In short, the zero tolerance hypothesis suggests that you would do best to give up alcohol altogether. Of course, abstinence will not prevent AIDS; however, it may delay the onset of AIDS as much as possible.

II. LEVELS OF DRINKING

A. ABSTINENCE
The first level of drinking is total abstinence or zero intake of alcoholic beverages. Sometimes abstinence is achieved by prohibition, but, when alcohol is denied, adults are strongly driven to find a way around the prohibition in order to get the product. This fact was clearly demonstrated during the Prohibition era in the United States. Specifically, adults will rebel if denied access to alcohol, and they will find a way to get around the authorities who make and enforce the laws prohibiting its production, distribution, and sale.

If an individual chooses abstinence for himself, especially for religious or sacred values, then he will likely be successful. For example, you might be sufficiently motivated to stop drinking in the face of death. On the other hand, various approaches taken by authority figures to force abstinence often meet with little or no success. Some of the familiar approaches include the statement, "It's not good for you", as well as threats, intimidation, laying blame, and physical abuse.

Abstinence fails when forced on persons who are not strongly committed to stop because it conflicts with powerful needs. One of these needs is to relax physically and mentally in order to temporarily escape from "reality". In this case, reality is one's perception of circumstance — degree of illness and closeness to death. You may desire to escape in order to stop thinking about AIDS and the prospect of death.

A second important need to drink alcohol is to facilitate social interactions in a group setting where drinking is customary behavior: "In most societies, drinking is a social act embedded in a context of values, attitudes, and other norms...."[2] This is true in the gay culture where bars constitute the general focus of social activities for many gays.[3] The bar is a place to meet friends and make new contacts in a "supportive" (i.e., gay) environment.

B. MODERATION
Moderate drinking constitutes the middle ground between abstinence and alcoholism. Probably the best description of moderate drinking is given in the 1990 edition of the "Dietary Guidelines" which states that an adult male may have no more than two drinks per day, and an adult female may have not more than one drink per day.[1] You may ask if you can save up your drinks and use them at the end of the week for a party or to go barhopping. The answer is no,

because one of the objectives of the guideline is to prevent excess intake on any single occasion. Additionally, as described below, binge drinking on weekends constitutes heavy drinking (Section II.C).

C. HEAVY INTAKE

It is difficult to pin down just what constitutes heavy use of alcoholic beverages. However, it is practical to suggest that it varies from 2 to 5 drinks per day for an adult male.[1,4] In this case, two drinks is consistent with moderate daily consumption as noted above (Section II.B) and five or more corresponds to alcoholism as discussed below (Section II.D). Heavy alcohol consumption is sometimes thought to be common among gay men.[3]

Alcohol may have taken up some of the slack created by the decreased use of other recreational drugs since the beginning of the AIDS epidemic. It is generally considered to be a desirable drug because it is a natural product closely linked to food. Additionally, it is legal, socially acceptable, and widely available at a low cost. There is a feeling that one can have a clear conscience when drinking alcohol.

Some HIV–positive gay men say they have given up other drugs and now alcohol is their only "vice". Apparently, alcohol is perceived as a minor threat to health. An important factor that might serve to rationalize this perception is its long history of safety as a food over thousands of years of use. In fact, the infected drinker may not "see" any ill effects of drinking; without some kind of physical sensation to serve as a warning, drinking behaviors are reinforced.

D. ALCOHOLISM

Alcoholism or alcohol abuse is defined as a pattern of alcohol use resulting in dysfunction in social settings or at work. The American Psychiatric Association classifies intake as: (1) regular heavy drinking, (2) heavy drinking on weekends, and (3) binges of drinking lasting for days, weeks, or months and separated by long periods of abstinence. A popular cutoff value for alcoholism was proposed by Vaillant[4] as five drinks per day.

III. ALCOHOL AND NUTRIENT INTAKE

A. OVERVIEW

Diet and nutritional status may be compromised in several ways by heavy or abusive alcohol consumption (Figure 3). Three important ways are (1) reduction of essential nutrient intakes from food by "empty" alcohol calories — the so–called "dilution" effect, (2) malabsorption of nutrients at the gut, and (3) unfavorable changes in the way nutrients are transported and stored within the body. Each of these leads to starvation at the tissue level where essential nutrients are used to build tissues or participate in other kinds of activities that promote the normal functioning of cells. In turn, this lack further compromises the immune system that is already damaged by the AIDS virus.

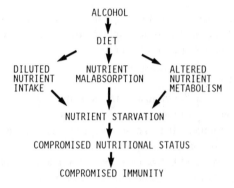

FIGURE 3.   Effects of alcohol on diet, nutritional status, and immunity.

B. FOOD CONSUMPTION

1. Empty Calories

Alcoholic beverages are generally considered to be "empty" calories. They do not make a significant contribution of any essential nutrients when consumed in normal amounts. Furthermore, these beverages do not provide the nutrients required for their complete metabolism at the liver. Thus, alcoholic beverage consumption places an added burden on the rest of the diet to provide not only for the body's needs, but also for the breakdown of alcohol. Nutrients particularly involved with the conversion of alcohol to energy include vitamins B_1 and B_2 biotin, niacin, pantothenic acid, magnesium, and zinc.

2. Diet Dilution

Alcoholic beverages are calorically rich, but nutrient poor. As their consumption goes up to a heavy level, they "displace" the intake of other, nutrient–dense foods. At this point, nutritionists say that the diet is "diluted" with alcohol calories because the relationship between energy and nutrients is shifted away from an incline with a positive slope toward one without a slope, the horizontal plot (Figure 4).

Figure 4 shows that iron intake increases as dietary energy intake increases. This same relationship exists for many other essential nutrients. If a nutrient were to plot in a horizontal fashion, then it could be concluded that it was present in only a few, select foods; the dietary intake level would be governed by a deliberate intake or failure to eat these foods.

Consider the situation where 100% of the energy intake comes from alcohol; no essential nutrients at all would be consumed because this source of calories is devoid of nutrients. To visualize this possibility, look at the flat, solid line at the zero (0) intake level of iron in Figure 4; this is a horizontal plot showing that nutrient intake is unrelated and does not increase regardless of the caloric value of alcoholic beverages consumed. Fortunately, "social" drinkers, those who imbibe moderately, do not have to worry about dilution or displacement of nutrient intakes because their intake is not sufficiently great. On the

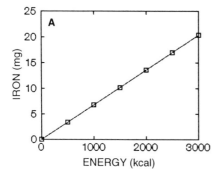
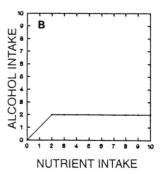

FIGURE 4. Actual and hypothetical relationships between dietary energy content and iron intake. Plot A: As caloric intake increases, so too does iron intake at a rate of about 6.8 milligrams per 1000 kcal (U.S. Department of Agriculture, 1984).[5] Plot B: With all energy coming from alcohol, there is no intake of essential nutrients, and the plot is horizontal.

other hand, alcoholics, those who drink very heavily on a daily basis, can and often do suffer from malnutrition leading to serious illness and death.

3. Hunger Suppression

Suppression of hunger is yet another way in which heavy alcohol consumption acts on nutritional status. In this case, the general desire to seek out and eat food is diminished, the intake of essential nutrients falls, and dietary quality suffers. Ironically, light alcohol consumption is well known to stimulate hunger, apparently by promoting relaxation.

C. NUTRIENT ABSORPTION

Alcohol is known to reduce the uptake of many nutrients from the gut. Some of these are vitamins A, D, E, and B complex; glucose; certain amino acids; zinc; sodium; magnesium; and calcium.[6] The malabsorption of nutrients that are chemically different and that differ widely in their mechanisms of absorption across the gut indicates alcohol must have a generalized effect on the gastrointestinal (GI) tract mucosa. One possibility is that alcohol causes general irritation or some kind of damage to the GI mucosa which disrupts the absorptive process.

D. NUTRIENT METABOLISM

For the purposes of this discussion, metabolism will be limited to the utilization of nutrients after they have been absorbed into the body, across the intestinal wall. Accordingly, alcohol impacts every phase of nutrient metabolism including distribution, activation, utilization, storage, degradation, and excretion.[7,8] Predictably, heavy alcohol use has negative consequences on both vitamins and minerals in relation to nutritional status. Deficiency and altered metabolism are especially prominent for vitamins B_1 and B_6 and folic acid. Persons with liver disease from long–term, heavy alcohol abuse show far more serious derangements of nutrient metabolism including failure to utilize amino acids to make sufficient quantities of blood proteins.

Water often does not get the attention it deserves in a nutritional context. Accordingly, alcohol is recognized as a diuretic; it increases urine formation and its elimination. In this regard, beer drinkers are familiar with the popular saying, "You can rent beer, but you can't buy it." Dehydration or water deficiency generally results from episodes of heavy drinking leading to shifts in the water content of body compartments, especially the blood and skeletal muscle tissue. Physical performance (exercise), body temperature regulation, and blood pressure are all adversely affected by dehydration (Chapter 3, Section IV.A.2.a). To correct dehydration, it is good to begin rehydration with nonalcoholic fluids as soon as possible, during or immediately after the episode.

E. NUTRIENT STARVATION AND IMMUNITY

When nutritional status is sufficiently compromised due to the effects of alcohol on nutrient intake, absorption, and metabolism, then the immune system becomes "starved" for nutrients (Chapter 1, Section I). It loses both readiness and responsiveness. In an HIV–infected person, this starvation further compromises an already damaged immune system because it needs all the nutrients it can get to keep fighting the primary HIV infection and any secondary opportunistic infections and to support the immune system. Starvation of essential nutrients further speeds the decline of the immune system, hastening the onset of AIDS, increasing the risk of opportunistic infections, and bringing about death faster than it would otherwise occur (Chapter 1, Section III.B).

IV. OTHER EFFECTS OF ALCOHOL

A. OVERVIEW

In addition to the effects of alcohol on nutritional status (Section III), it is relevant to consider its consequences for body tissues and the immune system. Alcohol is a nutrient in its own right, although not one that is required in the diet. These other effects should not be ignored because they are an important part of the total picture.

B. GENERAL IMMUNITY

Alcohol appears to create a disharmony among the various cellular components of the immune system in long–time alcoholics and experimental animals (Figure 5). The various components fall out of balance with one another. For example, the number of circulating T cells falls while the B cell count is unchanged. Imbalances might be explained by changes in the production rates of new cells for individual lymphocyte subpopulations. Additionally, alterations can occur in the "turnover" or "renewal" of individual lymphocyte subpopulations. The turnover process is characterized by a gradual replacement of

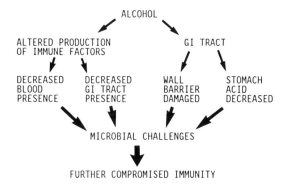

FIGURE 5. Effects of alcohol on production of immune factors (lymphocytes, antibodies, and immunoglobulins) and the gastrointestinal (GI) tract.

the cells within a given subpopulation where the time for renewal is dependent on what is needed to maintain a healthy state of readiness.

C. GASTROINTESTINAL TRACT INTEGRITY
1. Tract Wall

The GI tract begins at the mouth and continues down to the anus. This canal is continuously being subjected to microbes from food (Chapter 6, Section I). The first line of defense against invasion by foodborne organisms is a physical barrier — the wall of the GI tract itself. This wall is built of cells related to those making up your skin. Like skin, the cells of the GI tract are highly resistant to microbial invasion because they are tightly packed together so that there are no holes between them through which microbes can pass into the body from the canal.

Alcohol adversely affects the barrier function of the GI tract wall (Figure 5). Within minutes of consumption, it causes damage to the cells on the surface.[9] This compromises the integrity of the wall, allowing microbes to pass through it to the interior.

2. Acidic Stomach Contents

The second line of defense is the acidic stomach environment (Figure 5). The fluid in the stomach is always acidic, especially in the presence of food when microbes are likely to be present. The environment of the stomach is so harsh that nearly all microbes are killed in it. However, as discussed (Chapter 6), the stomach acid is only effective as long as the numbers of microbes present in meals are practical (i.e., typically low). Food that has been abused or otherwise contaminated can carry a very high load of microbes, and some will survive to move into the small intestine whether an individual is healthy or infected with HIV.

Chronic exposure to alcohol results in decreased production of acid in the stomach, and it becomes less acidic. Consequently, microbes survive when they should not. The stomach becomes a weak link in the chain of defense against microbes that are normally and unavoidably present in the food you eat. Microbes that would have been killed now move on into the small intestine where a nonacid (nearly neutral or slightly alkaline) environment permits them to thrive.

3. Immune Factors in the Gastrointestinal Tract

Immune factors such as immunoglobulins, particularly secretory IgA, are effective in killing microbes in the canal of the GI tract. They are active in the stomach and intestines, destroying viruses and fungi (bacteria, molds, and yeasts). HIV and other microbial challenges decrease the availability of these anti–infective factors by weakening the general immune system through changes in the production of immune factors (Figure 5). Consequently, there can be overgrowth of microbes normally present in the small intestine as well as those invading due to a breakdown of the GI tract barrier systems.

The surviving microbes change the makeup of the established and normal populations of microbes in the lower sections of the small intestine. There is a notable increase in organisms of fecal origin (coliforms); normally these microbes would be found only in the large intestine, where they are generally tolerated. When present in the small intestine, coliforms cause disease in man; normal gut activity would be disrupted and diarrhea might also result (Chapter 3).

With greater numbers of microbes in the small intestine, the probability increases that some will find a way to breach the intestinal wall. The resultant movement of microbes across the GI wall is likely to cause an infection in the bloodstream. This type of infection rapidly spreads to all body tissues as the blood is circulated.

Systemic (whole–body) infections can be very difficult to treat with conventional antibiotics in HIV–infected persons. For example, consider *Salmonella*, the pathogenic bacteria that is often found on the surface of poultry products. Because of compromised GI tract immunity, it takes fewer numbers of microbes to cause illness in the gut or body than it does in persons with an intact immune system. Once the organism gets established in the gut or body, the infected person is at a great disadvantage in mounting an effective challenge as compared with a well person. This is an important reason why the person with HIV infection must follow strict standards of sanitation when handling food and eating it (Chapter 6).

D. SPREAD OF HIV TO SUSCEPTIBLE TISSUES

It is important to recognize that HIV infection of the body does not occur in one sweeping takeover. Instead, the AIDS virus can invade only susceptible tissues throughout the body. This process takes place over a long period of time, depending on a variety of factors such as diet and nutritional status among others.

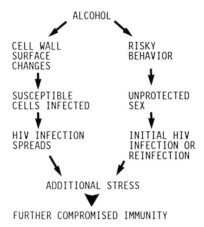

FIGURE 6. Dual effects of alcohol on the infection of HIV–susceptible tissue cells (marked with CD4 receptors) and risk–taking behavior.

HIV–susceptible tissues have cells with a specific marker on their surfaces; this marker is termed "CD4". Almost all popular attention has been focused on the T lymphocyte cells of the bloodstream as the target of HIV, but there are other tissue cells in the body with the CD4 receptor, including those of the skin, lung, brain, and GI tract. In time, all of these body tissues as well as others will become infected and dysfunctional, consistent with a diagnosis of AIDS.

A direct effect of alcohol for infected persons might be to speed up the rate of HIV infection throughout the body into susceptible tissues (Figure 6).[10] Alcohol has been shown to have an influence over the rate of infection of uninfected, but susceptible cells by the AIDS virus. Research with humans has demonstrated that cells of the immune system with the CD4 marker were infected by HIV more rapidly after the subjects drank alcoholic beverages. This result might be due to alcohol–induced damage to the exterior walls of susceptible cells so that they no longer function as effective barriers to HIV.

More importantly, these tests were conducted with humans drinking typical levels of alcohol intake, amounting to those found in 3 to 9 cans of beer (consumed in a single sitting). This preliminary work could have practical implications for persons who drink socially in moderate or heavy amounts.

These findings present a challenge to the traditional assumption that moderate drinking is without any negative consequence for health. Some scientists are now suggesting that even moderate drinking may be inappropriate given a condition of disease such as HIV infection. This suggests that abstinence is an option deserving serious consideration for persons with HIV infection.

E. RISK–TAKING BEHAVIORS

Alcohol surely provides a temporary escape from the constant awareness of HIV infection. It is a relief to push the threat of AIDS to the farthest reaches of the mind if only for a little while. At the same time, the anxieties associated with being infected are reduced, which may provide the freedom to talk about sex with prospective partners. This would be helpful if a frank exchange about HIV status were involved; however, there is some reason to believe that alcohol is also used for "courage" to engage in high–risk behaviors (i.e., unsafe or unprotected sex) (Figure 6).

HIV infection is still widely viewed as a terminal disease despite great advances in medicine. With this "death warrant", some who are infected figure that it is best to live to the fullest in the present. These persons give themselves a license to drink as much as they wish and may well engage in high–risk behaviors of many sorts, including binge drinking and alcoholism, both of which are immunosuppressive.

REFERENCES

1. Dietary Guidelines for Americans: Nutrition and Your Health, U.S. Department of Agriculture and U. S. Department of Health and Human Services, Washington, D.C., 1990.
2. National Research Council, *Diet and Health: Implications for Reducing Chronic Disease Risk*, National Academy Press, Washington, D.C., 1989, chap. 16.
3. **Martin, J. L.,** Drinking patterns and drinking problems in a community sample of gay men, in *Alcohol, Immunomodulation, and AIDS*, Seminara, D., Watson, R. R., and Pawlowski, A., Eds., Alan R. Liss, New York, 1990, 27.
4. **Vaillant, G. E.,** *The Natural History of Alcoholism*, Howard University, Washington, D.C., 1983.
5. Human Nutrition Information Service, *Nutrient Intake: Individuals in 48 States, Years 1977–78*, U.S. Dept. of Agriculture, Washington, D.C., 1984.

ADDITIONAL READING

Watson, R. R., Mohs, M. E., Eskelson, C., Sampliner R. E., and Hartmann, B., Identification of alcohol abuse and alcoholism with biological parameters, in *Alcoholism: Clin. Exp. Res.*, 10, 364, 1986.

Watson, R. R. and Leonard–Green, T. K., Alcohol–produced malnutrition and immunosuppression, in *Drugs of Abuse and Immune Function*, Watson, R. R., Ed., CRC Press, Boca Raton, FL, 1990, chap. 8.

Mohs, M. E. and Watson, R. R., Ethanol induced malnutrition, a potential cause of immunossuppression during AIDS, in *Alcohol, Immunomodulation, and AIDS*, Seminara, D., Watson, R. R., and Pawlowski, A., Eds., Alan R. Liss, New York, 1990, 433.

Kozol, R. A. and Elgebaly, S. A., Ethanol and its effects on mucosal immunity, in *Drugs of Abuse and Immune Function*, Watson, R. R., Ed., CRC Press, Boca Raton, FL, 1990, 19.

Watson, R. R., Immunomodulation by alcohol: a cofactor in development of AIDS after retrovirus infection, in *Cofactors in HIV–1 Infection and AIDS*, Watson, R. R., Ed., CRC Press, Boca Raton, FL, 1990, chap. 5.

Aldo–Benson, M., Ethanol and the B–cell: humoral immunity, in *Drugs of Abuse and Immune Function*, Watson, R. R., Ed., CRC Press, Boca Raton, FL, 1990, chap. 11.

Watson, R. R., Diagnosis of alcohol abuse by modulation of immune responses, in *Diagnosis of Alcohol Abuse*, Watson, R. R., Ed., CRC Press, Boca Raton, FL, 1989, chap. 6.

Watson, R. R. and Darban, H., Alcohol and immunosuppression, *Clin. Immunol.*, 9(8), 129, 1988.

Chapter 8

HIV–INFECTION IN WOMEN, INFANTS, AND CHILDREN

Saroj Bahl

CONTENTS

I. MAGNITUDE OF THE PROBLEM

Evidence accumulated in the last few years suggests that the incidence of HIV infection in women, infants, and children continues to increase. An examination of data from national mortality statistics reveals that the death rate for human immunodeficiency virus (HIV)/acquired immunodeficiency syndrome (AIDS) in women 15 to 44 years quadrupled between 1985 to 1988.[1] By 1987, HIV/AIDS had become one of the ten leading causes of death. Based on the current trends, HIV/AIDS may become one of the five leading causes of death in women of reproductive age in the 1990s.

The prevalence of HIV infection in children is also rising rapidly; it is anticipated that an additional 10,000 to 20,000 cases will be reported in the next few years.[2] This prediction is based on the continued increase of HIV infection in women of reproductive age. These women generally get infected from intravenous drug use with contaminated needles or infected sex partners. Once infected, they transmit the infection vertically to their infants. The majority of these infected infants will develop AIDS within the first 24 months of life, although some may remain asymptomatic for years.

A. IMPLICATIONS FOR THE HEALTH CARE SYSTEM

It is believed by several investigators that the actual prevalence of HIV infection in women, infants, and children may be underestimated. Several factors may be responsible for this low estimate. Patients or families may not wish to disclose their disease status due to ethical or legal problems. Also, because the primary source of pediatric AIDS is women of reproductive age, one has to consider the characteristics of this population. Most of these women are poor, have a minority status, and suffer from social isolation. To make matters worse, many are teenage mothers. Many of these women do not access the health care system due to cost, lack of transportation, and other psychosocial factors. Generally, HIV infection seems to predominate in the "no prenatal care" group.

One of the primary challenges confronting health care providers is outreach to the patients. Physicians and nurses should try to identify the various high–risk populations and initiate early diagnosis, treatment, and intervention. When financial and social resources are scanty, referral of the patient to other supportive services may be helpful.

B. CURRENT TREATMENT STRATEGIES

Complete cure of the disease is not presently available. The current treatment strategies are the same as for adult populations. The possibility of interrupting vertical transmission by administration of zidovudine (AZT) to HIV–infected pregnant women is being investigated by the AIDS Clinical Trials Group.[2] The potential for other antiviral investigational drugs in the treatment of pediatric AIDS is also being explored.

C. COST IMPLICATIONS

The cost of treating an HIV–infected infant on Medicaid has been estimated at $18,000 to $42,000. Health care costs for the management of women and children are similarly prohibitive. To complicate matters further, the disease seems to be predominantly confined to those who cannot afford it. Managing pediatric AIDS in a cost–effective manner is particularly a challenge because most cases come from socioeconomically disadvantaged families, where the mothers and sometimes even other family members are suffering from the illness.

II. TRANSMISSION OF HIV INFECTION FROM MOTHER TO INFANT

Almost all pediatric HIV infection can be attributed to maternal transmission of the viral infection to neonates. Hence, HIV infection in women is a primary cause of AIDS in the pediatric population. Although children comprise only 2% of the AIDS cases in the United States, the incidence of HIV infection in this population is rising rapidly. Several thousand additional cases are expected in the next few years. This increase will occur due to the increased number of women of reproductive age who will contract HIV infection. Because vertical transmission now accounts for more than 80% of AIDS cases in children under the age of 13, research efforts need to be concentrated on strategies for preventing this transfer.

A. RATE OF TRANSMISSION

Transmission of the infection from the mother to infant is relatively inefficient. Most studies have reported transmission rates of 20 to 30%; however, some investigators report a rate as high as 65%. It has been speculated that there may be a relationship between the stage of maternal illness and the rate of transmission. Studies conducted with women in Africa and France, which included cord blood cultures and CD4 assessment, indicated that women with advanced disease were more likely to transmit the infection to their infants.

B. MECHANISM OF TRANSMISSION

Passage of HIV infection from the mother to the fetus or newborn occurs *in utero;* however, the mechanism by which this transmission occurs is poorly understood. Suggestive evidence indicates that the transmission of infection may occur around the time of delivery. The virus has been identified in vaginal secretions. Nevertheless, some investigators have speculated that the virus may be transmitted through the placenta, perhaps early in the first trimester. The fetus may acquire the infection before the thymus achieves developmental maturity. This means that the fetus may contract HIV infection as much as 6 months before birth. Based on this information, it is not surprising that about 20% of the infected infants become symptomatic during the first few months of life. Further studies are necessary to elucidate the mechanism of transmission of HIV infection from mother to infant. This information, along with a determination of timing of transmission may assist in developing strategies for interrupting this process.

C. BREAST–FEEDING AND HIV TRANSMISSION

Studies indicate that women who are infected with HIV immediately post-partum (through blood transfusion) may transmit the infection to their infants through breast–feeding. Yet, others claim that infants who were breast–fed for as long as 7 months by women infected prepartum did not contract the HIV infection. Investigations in developing countries do not indicate increased rate of transmission by breast–feeding seropositive women in contrast to non-breast–feeding seropositive women; thus the risk of HIV transmission from breast–feeding is not well established. However, because HIV has been detected in lymphocytes in breast milk from seropositive mothers, breast–feeding is not recommended in developed countries including the United States.

III. PRENATAL CARE OF HIV–INFECTED WOMEN INCLUDING NUTRITIONAL MANAGEMENT

A. PRENATAL CARE

The prevalence of HIV infection is high among the minority ethnic/racial groups and low–income families. Several HIV–infected mothers–to–be from these families may not seek prenatal care until late in their pregnancies. Many factors may contribute to the late entry of these women into the health care system, including poverty, social isolation, minority status, and alienation. Yet, the beneficial effect of comprehensive prenatal care on the outcome of a pregnancy is well documented. It has also been shown that HIV–infected women are more likely to give birth to premature, low birth weight, and malnourished infants. Prenatal care, including nutrition intervention, may possibly reduce these poor outcomes.

Thus, health care providers should make a concerted effort to make prenatal care available to these needy clients. These underprivileged individuals cannot afford private health insurance; cost remains a factor in the denial of health services. However, studies indicate that women will seek prenatal health care as long as it is of good quality, accessible, and affordable.

B. NUTRITIONAL MANAGEMENT

It is well recognized that the course and outcome of a normal, uncomplicated pregnancy is significantly affected by the nutritional status of the mother. In the HIV–infected pregnancy, the role of nutrition becomes even more crucial. The serious and chronic nature of this viral infection necessitates an enhanced need for calories, protein, and other essential nutrients created by the state of physiological stress. Pregnancy itself is an anabolic state and requires calories, protein, and nutrients over and above the nonpregnant state. A combination of these factors translates to considerably higher nutrient requirements for the HIV–infected woman. Since nutritional intake in pregnancy is affected by many physical and psychosocial factors, a personalized dietary/nutritional care plan needs to be designed to meet the specific needs of the HIV–infected pregnant woman.

1. Nutritional Assessment

The first step in the creation of a nutritional care plan is assessment of nutritional status. This requires collection of information related to the patient's medical history, anthropometric measurements, physical examination, and several biochemical tests. A dietary history should also be obtained. These categories including several essential components are presented in Table 1.

Collection of this information is helpful because it may provide essential baseline data for nutritional planning. For example, when a pregnant women is underweight at the start of the pregnancy, she may need special intervention. Her requirements for energy would need to be adjusted to permit weight gain additional to that required in a normal pregnancy. It also needs to be remembered that HIV infection itself, particularly in the advanced stage, is a progressive catabolic disorder characterized by severe weight loss.

Information related to psychosocial factors, such as low socioeconomic status and lack of family or social support, is also helpful because it may identify the need for community and social service. Low levels of serum albumin, hematocrit, etc. may indicate increased need for protein, iron, and other essential nutrients. Hence, the vital importance of nutritional assessment of HIV–infected pregnant women cannot be overemphasized.

TABLE 1
Parameters Used for Evaluation of Nutritional Status
in HIV–Infected Pregnant Women

Various components of nutrition assessment

Anthropometric measurements
   Weight
   Height
   Midarm circumference
   Triceps skinfold thickness

Biochemical tests
   Hemoglobin levels
   Hematocrit
   Serum albumin
   Total protein

Physical examination
   Signs of malnutrition
   Color of skin, nails, etc.

Dietary history
   24–hour recall
   Food frequency

Medical history
   Previous obstetric history
   Presence of chronic disease
   Gestational diabetes

2. Estimation of Energy and Protein Requirements

Energy requirements for pregnant women are significantly higher due to the metabolic demands of pregnancy and fetal growth. The Recommended Dietary Allowances (RDA) established by the Food and Nutrition Board of the National Research Council/National Academy of Sciences (NRC/NAS) suggest an additional allowance of 300 kcal above the nonpregnant energy needs. It is difficult, though, to quantify energy needs for individual women. Factors such as prepregnancy weight, stage of pregnancy, and level of physical activity may influence the actual energy needs.

The nutritional needs of HIV–infected pregnant women have not been determined. One can only speculate on this issue or apply the knowledge gained from other similar situations. HIV infection is a serious chronic infection characterized by hypermetabolism, malabsorption, negative nitrogen balance, and malnutrition. Like other chronic infections, nutritional management may necessitate a generous energy and protein allowance. The daily energy and protein needs are likely to be very high due to the combined demands placed on the woman by her state of pregnancy and HIV infection. Energy needs for most women may be in the range of 2400 to 3000 kcal.

The current RDA for protein is 60 grams for normal pregnancy; again, the requirement for this nutrient may be significantly higher for HIV–infected women. Energy and protein requirements are hard to separate. When energy intake is insufficient to meet the bodily needs, protein is catabolized to release energy. It is difficult to distinguish between the effects of energy and protein deficiency. Results of some studies have shown that the provision of extra energy has the same favorable effect on the outcome of pregnancy as providing protein and energy together.[3] From these findings, it appears that usually the energy deficit and not the protein deficit determines the outcome of a pregnancy.

3. Prenatal Weight Gain

Adequacy of energy and protein intake is reflected in the pattern of prenatal weight gain. Because optimum requirements of energy and protein cannot be accurately ascertained in a normal or complicated pregnancy, the most appropriate approach is to monitor the weight gain regularly. The NAS recommends a weight gain of 25 to 35 pounds for women of normal weight, 28 to 40 pounds for underweight women, and 15 to 25 pounds for overweight women (Figure 1).

Achieving an adequate pattern of weight gain in the HIV–complicated pregnancy represents a complex challenge. The presence of diarrhea, malabsorption, and opportunistic infections may make it difficult to gain weight. Devising a nutritional care plan that includes a patient's likes and dislikes, suggestions for resolving nutrition–related problems, and provision of emotional and psychosocial support may be helpful to the patient. In cases of extreme nausea, vomiting, and inadequate weight gain or continued weight loss, alternate means of nutritional support such as enteral or parenteral feeding may become necessary.

4. Vitamin and Mineral Needs

Requirements for most vitamins and minerals are significantly increased during pregnancy. The presence of chronic infection also enhances the need for certain vitamins. Although research on vitamin and mineral needs in HIV infection has not been conducted yet, one can assume that the situation is similar to other chronic infections. Together, these factors translate to higher needs for these nutrients in the HIV–infected pregnant woman.

Requirements for several vitamins — pyridoxine (B_6), folacin, cobalamin (B_{12}), D, E, and C — are known to increase during normal pregnancy. Similarly, the daily needs for several minerals — zinc, iron, magnesium, calcium, phosphorus, iodine, and selenium — are enhanced. Expansion of blood volume, red blood cell production, and rapid cell proliferation in the maternal and fetal tissues (all physiological changes) necessitate increased amounts of iron, folate, vitamin B_{12}, and zinc in the mother's diet. Several of these nutrients are not obtained easily either because of their limited availability in food sources or because of poor food choices made by the mother. Supplements of vitamins and minerals may become necessary.

Several types of prenatal vitamin and mineral supplements are available; these could be selected and prescribed after a personalized analysis of the pregnant woman's current diet has been conducted. Chronic infections such as tuberculosis are known to be associated with an increased need for several

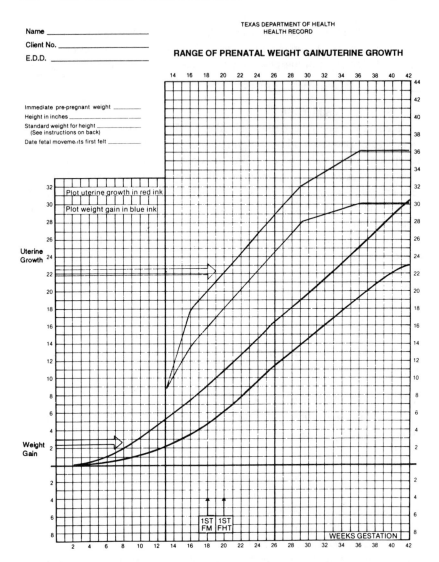

FIGURE 1.   Prenatal weight gain grid that demonstrates desirable weight gain ranges for normal pregnant women. (Developed by Texas Department of Health; Austin, Texas.)

nutrients, particularly protein and vitamins A and C. A similar situation may exist in HIV infection; however, further research is needed in these areas. Until then, it would be prudent to follow the recommendations for a normal pregnancy. Physicians, nurses, and dietitians should monitor the patient's eating habits and nutritional intake and prescribe appropriate supplements as necessary.

5. Opportunistic Infections

In HIV–infected individuals, immune dysfunction may occur long before clinical manifestations appear. This makes the patient very prone to several opportunistic infections. Because the state of pregnancy itself is a period of physiological stress, it may also increase the vulnerability of the pregnant woman to infections. It is known that several hormones produced during pregnancy may suppress some components of the immunologic system such as the lymphocytes. If malnutrition is superimposed on one or both of these conditions, the situation is further aggravated. Adequate therapy of the opportunistic infections, nutritional management of drug–induced side effects (see Chapter 5), treatment of oral and gastrointestinal complications when they exist (see Chapter 4), and following general guidelines for a balanced and good quality diet are essential components of nutritional intervention.

6. Individualized Dietary Counseling

A pregnant woman is highly motivated toward taking care of her health at this time of her life because she knows that her health and nutritional status may have a direct bearing on her infant. Most women are willing to abstain from alcohol, smoking, and drugs, as well as pay special attention to their food habits. Health professionals, dietitians, and caregivers should take advantage of this opportune time to counsel the patient regarding the benefits of a nutritious diet and a healthy lifestyle. A dietitian's role involves planning an adequate dietary prescription that takes the pregnant client's food preferences and aversions into consideration. As a pregnant woman starts adhering to the diet, her health will improve and this will improve compliance.

IV. HIV INFECTION AND AIDS IN THE PEDIATRIC POPULATION

A. MORBIDITY AND MORTALITY

The proportion of pediatric AIDS has remained fairly constant since 1983, when it was first reported. Of the 41,825 cases of AIDS reported to Centers for Disease Control (CDC) in 1987, 609 (1.5%) were pediatric patients. These cases have been confined to infants and children under 13 years of age. Reported overall, mortality rates have ranged from 57 to 73%. The majority of the patients acquired the disease perinatally.

Most of these patients develop clinical illness within the first 24 months of life even though they appear normal and asymptomatic at birth. Acute respiratory failure (ARF), associated with opportunistic infections, is the most common cause of death in the majority of the pediatric patients. Several of these patients are hospitalized in a pediatric intensive care unit (PICU) at least once during their lifetime.[3] The extremely high morbidity and mortality associated with pediatric AIDS is likely to have a strong impact on health care resources.

B. TYPES OF PEDIATRIC AIDS

Pediatric AIDS can be congenital, that is, acquired through vertical transmission from an HIV–infected mother, or it may be transmitted through transfusions of blood and blood products. About 20% of the cases fall in the latter category. Due to the thorough screening measures instituted since 1985, these sources have been almost eliminated. However, HIV infection in the latter category can take 3 to 10 years to develop. Thus, new cases continue to be identifed.

Pediatric AIDS may follow one of two courses: early onset disease and late onset. In the early onset type, severe immunodeficiency occurs rather rapidly in the first year of life. In this type of population, the most common illness is Pneumocystis carinii pneumonia (PCP), and it is usually fatal. In the late onset HIV infection, some children may remain asymptomatic for years. Then they may exhibit a number of clinical manifestations. These are summarized in the next section.

C. CLINICAL FEATURES

As stated earlier, the majority of HIV–infected infants may develop clinical symptoms within the first 24 months of life. Some, however, may remain asymptomatic for as many as 8 years. The progression from the asymptomatic to the symptomatic stage in infants may have a rather rapid onset.

HIV infection in infants is associated with several serious clinical manifestations, such as failure to thrive, chronic/recurrent diarrhea, enlargement of the liver and spleen (hepatosplenomegaly), and inflammation of parotid glands and lymph nodes (parotitis and lymphadenopathy). Like adults, they may also suffer from several opportunistic infections such as PCP, oral and esophageal candidiasis, and several recurrent bacterial infections.

There are several distinguishing clinical features between HIV infection in children and adults. These are summarized in Table 2.

As indicated, children are more susceptible to recurrent bacterial infections, cytomegalovirus infections, chronic swelling/inflammation of the parotid gland, and cases of lymphoid interstitial pneumonitis (LIP). On the other hand, B cell lymphoma and Kaposi's sarcoma, which are commonly observed in adults, rarely occur in children. Neurological problems associated with HIV infection of the central nervous system are more frequent in children.

D. TREATMENT

In 1990, the drug zidovudine (AZT) was approved for therapy of HIV infection in children. In 1981, studies indicated that the progression of HIV infection to AIDS in asymptomatic or minimally symptomatic adults could be delayed by the administration of zidovudine, particularly if the drug was given

TABLE 2
Distinguishing Clinical Features Between Pediatric and Adult AIDS

Clinical feature	Pediatric population	Adult population
Weight loss	More significant clinically; failure to thrive present in 94% cases	Occurs more during advanced stages; can be controlled more easily than in pediatric patients
Opportunistic infections	Bacterial infections occur more frequently; LIP occurs more commonly	Viral and bacterial infections occur; PCP can occur but prophylaxis can delay it
Kaposi's sarcoma and B cell lymphoma	Occurs rarely in children	Occurs often in adults
Neurological dysfunctioning	More pronounced in children	Occurs but less often

when the CD4 count fell below 500. One could assume that possibly the same effect would occur if the drug was administered to children. The Food and Drug Administration recommends that in infants evidence of compromised immunologic function instead of a precise CD4 count should be taken as an indicator for initiation of therapy. The levels of CD4 are not the only criterion for antiviral therapy; other parameters such as hypergammaglobulinemia may also be used.[2] Although zidovudine has been shown to be somewhat effective in infants and children and is also generally well tolerated, other forms of antiviral therapy are desperately needed. Preliminary results with administration of intravenous gammaglobulin have shown some promise. The normal vaccination schedule should still be followed in HIV–infected infants; in fact, special attention should be given to vaccines against two diseases — polio and measles.

E. NUTRITIONAL MANAGEMENT

Infancy and childhood are characterized by a very rapid rate of growth. Normal infants triple their birth weight at the end of the first year. This rapid rate of physical growth and development necessitates adequate nutritional support. Infection with HIV superimposes a state of chronic stress on a highly anabolic, tissue–building phase of life. The importance of nutritional management is self–evident.

1. Assessment of Growth and Nutrition

Some studies indicate that poor growth and failure to thrive (FTT) are present in 94% of the pediatric patients.[4] HIV–infected infants may not demonstrate any weight gain initially. If the patient becomes symptomatic, weight loss may even occur. This may be caused by increased nutrient losses, malabsorption, and elevated metabolic needs due to infection and fever. Need for calories, protein, vitamins, and minerals is enhanced significantly in this state. The primary objective of nutritional management is to prevent weight loss and promote normal gains in weight.

The most appropriate approach for ascertaining nutritional adequacy of food intake in infants and children is by assessment of growth and nutritional status. This should include several essential parameters that are summarized in Table 3.

Growth in infants and children is assessed by plotting their weight and height on standardized growth curves. The most commonly used growth curves are those developed by the National Center for Health Statistics (NCHS). Two age groups are available — birth to 36 months and 2 through 18 years. The curves include weight and height–for–age as well as weight–for–height. An infant or child who falls below the fifth percentile for weight and/or height is classified as FTT. On these growth curves, normal healthy children should fall between the 25th and 75th percentile, with the average weight being around the 50th percentile. In addition to physical growth, other anthropometric parameters such as triceps skinfold, midarm circumference, midarm muscle circumference, head circumference, etc. should be assessed (Figures 2 through 5).

Regular evaluation of biochemical parameters such as serum albumin, total iron–binding capacity, blood urea nitrogen (BUN), creatinine, serum potassium, and complete blood count should also be conducted. In addition, tests of hepatic and kidney function should be performed regularly. Caregivers and dietitians should monitor the infants/child's appetite and food intake. Tolerance of the food and feeding strategies should also be assessed regularly.

2. Determination of Energy and Protein Requirements

Data related to protein and energy requirements of HIV–infected infants and children are very scarce. Some investigators have recommended the use of RDA plus an allowance for stress, suggesting using the weight at the 50th percentile as an ideal body weight (for the corresponding age or height).[5] Others recommend using 100 kcal/kg for the first 10 kg of body weight, 50 kcal/kg for the second 10 kg, and 20 kcal/kg for each kg over 20 kg of body weight.[5] Most agree that additional calories must be calculated and provided for fever, infection, and associated illness. The most appropriate technique for assessing caloric and nutrient adequacy, as stated earlier, is regular monitoring of weight. Weekly assessment of weight gain is necessary because this may serve as an indicator for caloric adjustments.

Typically, protein requirements for infants and young children are based on their weight in kilograms. It has been recommended that these requirements should be increased by 50 to 100% to compensate for loss of nitrogen and increased metabolic needs. Requirements for protein should always be

TABLE 3
Assessment of Growth and Nutrition in HIV–Infected Children

Assessment parameters

Physical growth/anthropometrics	Biochemical tests
Weight for age and height	Serum albumin
Height–for–age	Total iron binding capacity (TIBC)
Head circumference	Total blood count
Triceps skinfold	Blood urea nitrogen (BUN)
Midarm circumference	Creatinine
Midarm muscle circumference	Liver function tests

Diet history
Tolerance to food
24–hour recall
Food frequency
Snacking patterns

considered along with caloric needs; deficiency of one affects the other. These requirements may increase during phases of "catch–up" growth, for example, when the pediatric patient has just recovered from an acute illness and is trying to compensate for normally anticipated but missed weight gains.

Energy and protein requirements for normal children are calculated by a variety of formulas; there is no agreement on a particular method. The situation is further complicated in HIV–infected pediatric patients because we are dealing with a chronic infection for which the etiology, mechanism of disease production, etc. are poorly understood. Nevertheless, it is well known that the needs for protein and energy are significantly increased. Hence, once again, the best strategy is growth assessment. Each patient serves as his/her own control; whatever energy intake promotes an adequate growth rate in that particular individual is the best calculated caloric level. During acute infection, though, maintenance of weight gain may be a more realistic objective than weight gain.

3. Guidelines for Feeding HIV–Infected Infants and Children

As stated earlier, breast–feeding by HIV–infected women should be contraindicated in the United States and other developed countries to avoid that possible route of HIV infection. Bottle–feeding, using a milk–based formula, is the alternative method of feeding infants. The caloric density of the formula can be increased by adding Polycose® (glucose polymer), medium chain trig-lycerides (MCT), or vegetable oil (safflower or corn oil). Adjustments should be made in the dosage, source, caloric density, and timing schedule of the formula as needed based on the infant's tolerance of the feeding.

Children should be fed a normal, well–balanced diet; however, special consideration should be given to inclusion of high–energy, nutrient–dense

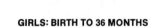

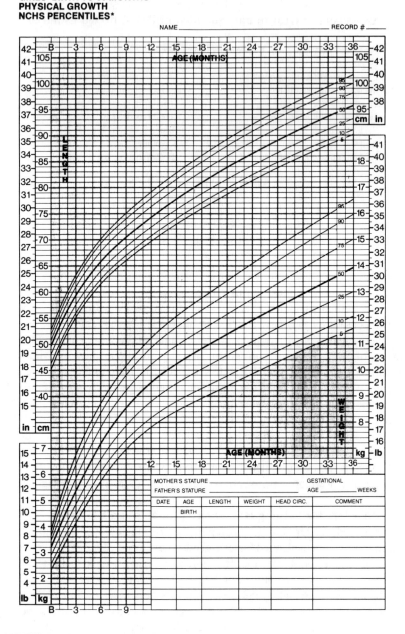

FIGURE 2. Growth curves for girls — birth to 36 months. (Used with permission of Ross Products Division, Abbott Laboratories; Columbus, Ohio 43216. From NCHS Growth Charts ©1982; Ross Products Division, Abbott Laboratories.)

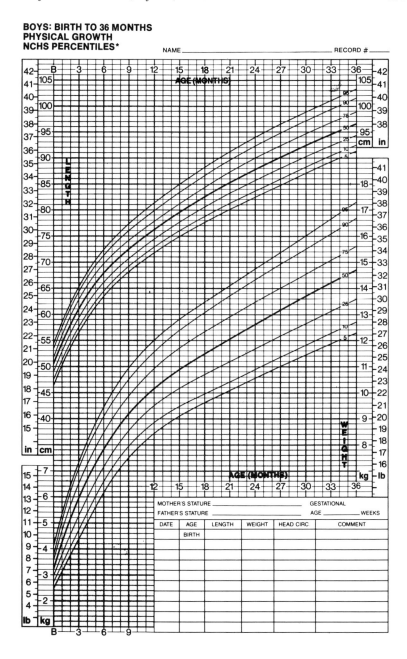

FIGURE 3. Growth curves for boys — birth to 36 months. (Used with permission of Ross Products Division, Abbott Laboratories; Columbus, Ohio 43216. From NCHS Growth Charts ©1982; Ross Products Division, Abbott Laboratories.)

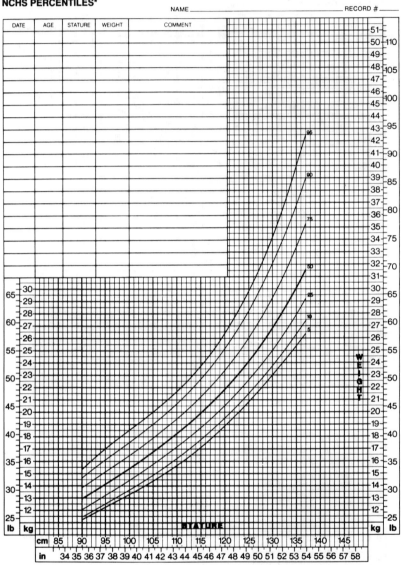

FIGURE 4.   Growth curves for girls — prepubescent 2 to 18 years. (Used with permission of Ross Products Division, Abbott Laboratories; Columbus, Ohio, 43216. From NCHS Growth Charts ©1982; Ross Products Division, Abbott Laboratories.)

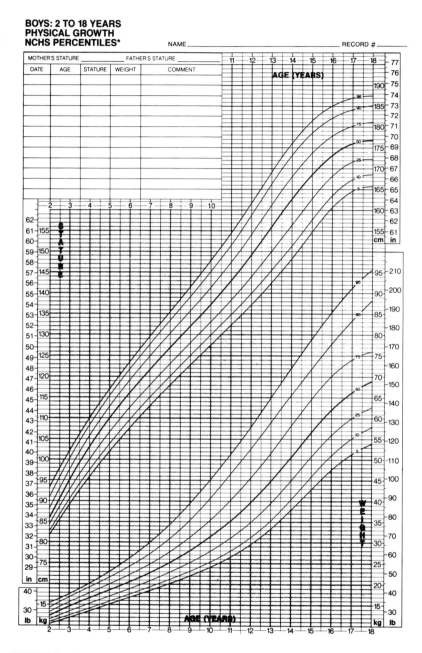

FIGURE 5. Growth curves for boys — prepubescent 2 to 18 years. (Used with permission of Ross Products Division, Abbott Laboratories; Columbus, Ohio 43216. From NCHS Growth Charts ®1982; Ross Products Division, Abbott Laboratories.)

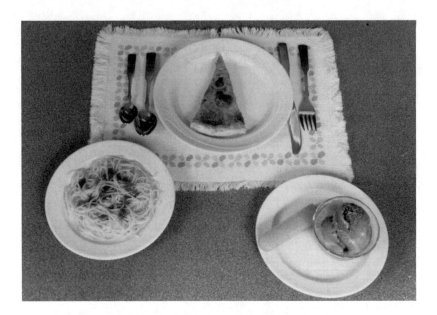

FIGURE 6.   Foods that are special favorites of children should be served. Theses include ice cream, pizza, pasta with mild seasoning, Popsicles®, etc.

feedings. Small, more frequent meals are good general recommendations for both infants and children. Particular attention should be given to children's likes and dislikes; foods that are special favorites should be provided more frequently. These may include foods such as ice cream, milk shakes, desserts, pizza, creamy pasta with mild seasoning, buttered sauces and gravies, casseroles, etc. (Figure 6). In addition, special attention should be given to food safety and food service types of issues (see Chapter 6).

4. Nutritional Problems Associated with Malnutrition

Due to the heavy demands of rapid growth in infants and young children, as well as the hypermetabolic nature of HIV infection, these populations are particularly prone to developing clinical manifestations of malnutrition. It is essential to recognize the various types of problems that may lead to malnutrition and resolve them with appropriate nutritional strategies.

a. Poor Food Intake

Poor appetite and consequently decreased food intake may be associated with infections, fever, side effects of medications, or emotional factors. Chewing, sucking, and swallowing may become extremely painful and difficult activities due to the presence of oral and esophageal infections. Strategies to overcome such problems with modifications of food have been discussed in Chapter 4. These may need to be adjusted for infants and children. For example, infants who have sucking problems due to the presence of mouth ulcers and sores may need to be fed with spoons or medicine droppers. Feeding of such infants may require considerable time, effort, and patience. For older children with similar problems, soft, mildly seasoned, and nonspicy foods such as creamed soups, scrambled eggs, ice cream, cooked cereals, etc. can be given. Acidic, rough, and spicy foods should be omitted.

b. Developmental Delay

As stated earlier, neurological dysfunction is more common in HIV–infected pediatric patients in contrast to adults. This may delay the appearance of developmental milestones in infants and children. Development of normal feeding skills may not follow the predicted progression. Older children, 3 to 4 years old, may require bottle–feeding. Adaptations of usual feeding techniques to match the patient's needs may become essential.

c. Opportunistic Infections

Like adults, HIV–infected infants and children may be very prone to developing several opportunistic infections. The situation is aggravated by the fact that the immune system is not well developed in these age groups. Gastrointestinal infections such as atypical myobacterium, cytomegalovirus, and cryptosporidium may cause severe diarrhea in the pediatric population. Fever, weight loss, and malabsorption that accompany these opportunistic infections further aggravate the resultant malnutrition as well as the immunocompromised state. Special nutritional management strategies may become essential, such as increasing intake of calories and protein, lactose restriction, elemental diets, and supplementation with vitamins and minerals. Supplemental or total nutritional support can be provided through tube feeding. Parenteral nutrition may be used as needed.

d. Respiratory Problems

The occurrence of respiratory problems is very common in the pediatric population. As mentioned earlier, a majority of pediatric patients die of acute respiratory failure (ARF) secondary to opportunistic infections. Respiratory problems that occur in the pediatric population include PCP, desquamative interstitial pneumonia (DIP), and lymphoid interstitial pneumonia (LIP). These are accompanied by labored breathing and a rapid respiratory rate which necessitate increased intake of calories.

5. Nutrient Deficiencies and Their Correction

HIV infection is likely to be associated with several nutrient deficiencies, because the needs for some nutrients may be higher due to the hypermetabolism evident in this infection as well as excessive losses. For example, zinc may be lost in excessive amounts in urine and sweat. Folate deficiency has been associated with neurological degeneration; development of cardiomyopathy may be related to selenium deficiency. Hence, supplemental vitamins and minerals, one or two times the RDA, may be beneficial. Excessive amounts of some minerals such as zinc and iron should be contraindicated due to possible adverse effects on the immune system.

6. Aggressive Nutritional Support

Whenever possible, oral feeding should be encouraged in pediatric patients. However, in cases of weight loss, severe anorexia, and malnutrition associated with poor intake, alternative methods of nutritional support are well justified.

Oral intake can be supplemented with additional nutritional support through tube feedings. If the gastrointestinal tract is functioning, a nasoenteric tube feeding can be used. In the case of severe discomfort due to oral and gastrointestinal lesions, parenteral nutrition may become necessary. However, one has to carefully weigh the potential benefits vs. risks. It is well known that total parenteral nutrition (TPN) is associated with catheter–related complications. Liver damage has been attributed to long–term TPN usage. It is perhaps better to use TPN on a short–term basis and to resort to it only when absolutely necessary.

Improving the overall health and quality of life is the goal of all nutritional interventions. Each patient may have a unique situation and may demonstrate a different response to various forms of nutritional support than another case. Hence, each individual's tolerance to a certain form of feeding should be evaluated carefully. Accordingly, different approaches of feeding should be selected.

V. HIV INFECTION IN ADOLESCENTS

The transmission of HIV infection to adolescents occurs by the same routes as in adults. Approximately 1% of the AIDS cases occur in this population. The most common mode of HIV transmission in teen years is through sexual activity. Clinical manifestations and management of HIV infection in this population are very similar to adults.

VI. PREVENTIVE STRATEGIES

HIV infection/AIDS is a fatal disease. The fact that this devastating disease has also affected women of child–bearing age, infants, and children is an alarming issue. While efforts are constantly being made in the direction of a cure, prevention of the spread of this disease needs to become a public health priority. Particular attention needs to be directed toward the high–risk populations — the low–income, minority status women in whom the infection appears to have a high prevalence. Concerted efforts are now required of health care professionals, caregivers, and the community for embarking on a comprehensive health educational program that emphasizes the importance of prevention.

This philosophy is no different than that emphasized for other chronic, degenerative, and ultimately fatal diseases such as cardiovascular disease, cancer, hypertension, etc. where prevention is better than cure.

REFERENCES

1. **Chu, S. Y., Buehler, J. W., and Berkelman, R. L.,** Impact of the human immunodeficiency virus epidemic on mortality in women of reproductive age, United States, *Am. Med. Assoc.,* 264(2), 225, 1990.
2. **Wilfert, C. M.,** HIV infection in maternal and pediatric patients, *Hosp. Pract.,* 26(5), 55, 1991.
3. **Wilkinson, J. D., and Greenwald, B. M.,** The acquired immunodeficiency syndrome: impact on the pediatric intensive care unit, *Crit. Care Clin.,* 4(4), 831, 1988.
4. **Shannon, K. M., and Ammann, A. J.,** Acquired immune deficiency syndrome in childhood, *J. Pediatr.,* 106(2), 332, 1985.
5. **Bentler, M., and Stanish, M.,** Nutrition support of the pediatric patients with AIDS, *J. Am. Diet. Assoc.,* 87(4), 488, 1987.
6. **Mugrditchian, L., Arent–Fine, J., and Dwyer, J.,** The nutrition of the HIV–infected child. Part I. A review of clinical issues and therapeutic strategies, *Top. Clin. Nutr.,* 7(2), 1, 1992.
7. **Oleske, J. M., Connor, E. M., Grebenau, M. D., and Minnefor, A. B.,** Treatment of HIV–infected infants and children, *Pediatr. Ann.,* 17(5), 334, 1988.
8. Task Force on Pediatric AIDS, Perinatal human immunodeficiency virus infection, *Pediatrics,* 82(6), 941, 1988.
9. Special Medical Reports, AAP issues statement on perinatal HIV infection, *Am. Fam. Physician,* 39(3), 390, 1989.
10. **Mahan, L. K., and Arlin, M.,** *Krause's Food, Nutrition and Diet Therapy,* 8th ed., W. B. Saunders, Philadelphia, 1992, chaps. 9 and 37.

INDEX

A

abdominal distention, 81

abdominal pain, 55, 76

    from opportunistic infections, 81, 82, 103

    as symptom of foodborne illness, 135

absorption of vitamins and minerals, 32, 34, 42, 153. *See also* malabsorption

abstinence from alcohol, 150

acid indigestion, 54, 57–58, 72

acidity, and microbial growth in food, 124, 125

acid secretions from stomach, 6, 155–156

acute necrotizing ulcerative gingivitis, 91. *See also* gingivitis

acute respiratory failure (ARF), 177

acyclovir, 102

    for *Candidiasis*, 80

    for viral infections, 81, 82, 100, 103, 105

adipose tissue, 59

adolescents, HIV infection in, 178

adrenal insufficiency, 41, 80

age, and energy expenditure, 22

AIDS

    definition, 38

    drug therapies for, 98–102

    predisposing factors, 9–11

    symptom progression towards, 10–11, 40, 55, 80, 96–97, 102

    weight loss during, compared with other diseases, 42–43

AIDS Clinical Trials Group, 161

AIDS enteropathy, 55

albumin, 48, 92

alcohol, 148–158

    USDA dietary guidelines for, 14, 20, 148–149

alcoholism, 20, 151

algae, classification of, 118, 134

allergies to food, 79, 84

alternative medical therapies, 97

alveolar bone, 84

American Dietetic Association, 112

amino acids, 153, 154

amphotericin B, 80, 103, 106, 112

anemia, 5, 99, 106, 112

angular cheilitis, 77

animals in nutritional research, 4

anorexia, 15, 18, 23–24, 76

    causes of, 40

    as a drug side effect, 104

    overcoming, 28–30

    and protein intake, 31

antacids, excessive use of, 54, 57–58, 72

anthropometric measurements, 91–92

antibiotics, prolonged use of, 54, 57

antibody response, 5, 9

antifungal medications, 78, 80, 106

antioxidants, 8

antiviral medications, 48, 81, 82, 97, 99–102

anxiety, 40–41

appetite stimulants, 48

appetite suppression, 47, 153, 176–177

ARF (acute respiratory failure), 177

ascorbic acid. *See* vitamin C

aspiration (feeding problem), 77

atrophic candidiasis, 77, 79

autoimmune effects, 102

azidothymidine. *See* zidovudine

AZT. *See* zidovudine

B

"background noise", in monitoring body weight, 25, 26

bacon, 29

bacteria

    classification of, 118, 134

    and food sanitation, 71–72, 116–146

    and food water activity scores, 120

bacterial infections, 43, 79, 83, 168

bactericidal secretions from skin, 6

Bactrim™, 104, 107

balance beam scales, 25–26

barrier integrity, 6

    blood-brain, 101

    of gastrointestinal tract lining, 4, 5–6, 7, 117, 155–156

    of skin, 4, 5

"basic four food groups", 14, 15, 16, 19

bathroom scales, 25

B cell antibodies, 97

    effect of alcohol on, 154–155

B cell lymphoma, 168, 169

BCM (body cell mass), 23, 40

beans, 12

polyunsaturated fatty acids, 8
Popsicles®, 85
pork, 16–17
potassium. *See also* sodium
  in blood, 170
  depletion as a drug side effect, 103
  depletion during chronic diarrhea, 40,
    61–62
  in juice, 63
potatoes, 29
poultry, 16–17, 136
predisposing factors in AIDS, 9–11
pregnancy, 161, 162–167
prenatal care of HIV-infected women,
    162–167
prenatal weight gain, 165, 166
prevention of weight loss, 47–49
progestins, for anorexia management, 48
prophylaxis, 104–105
propionic acid, and microbial growth in
    foods, 124, 142
protein, 15, 16–17
  conversion to glucose, 44
  depletion during chronic diarrhea, 59
  synthesis, 6
protein-calorie malnutrition (PCM), 38, 40,
    42, 45
protein intake, 30–31
  decrease by alcohol use, 151–154
  estimating requirements, 45–46
  recommended dietary allowances of, 30,
    164
  requirements of HIV-infected children
    and infants, 170–171
  requirements of pregnant women,
    164–165
proteolysis, 44
protozoal infections, 78, 82, 106–107
protozoans, classification of, 118, 134
pseudomembranous candidiasis, 77, 80
Pseudomonas, 121
psychological factors, 163
  of anorexia, 40–41
  during chronic diarrhea, 53
  during oral and esophageal complications,
    92
psyllium, 66–67
pyrazinamide, 103, 112
pyridoxine. *See* vitamin B$_6$
pyrimethamine, 103

R

radiation therapy, 83
radicals (oxygen), 8
rashes, as a drug side effect, 102, 103, 104
RAU (recurrent aphthous ulcers), 84
raw milk, 142–143
reading labels, 12
recommended dietary allowances (RDA),
    19, 30, 31, 33–34, 164
  in HIV-infected infants and children, 178
recurrent aphthous ulcers (RAU), 84
refrigeration of food, 121–123, 131
renal dysfunction, 112
renal toxicity, 47, 103, 104, 107
respiratory problems, in HIV-infected
    infants and children, 177
restaurant eating, 141–143
retinol. *See* vitamin A
retinol-binding protein, 92
retrosternal pain, 80
Retrovir therapy, 41
reverse transcripterase, 99, 100
riboflavin. *See* vitamin B$_2$
ribonucleic acid (RNA), 6, 7
rifampin, 103
risk-taking behaviors, and alcohol, 157–158
RNA (ribonucleic acid), 6, 7
rodents, 133

S

saliva, enzyme secretions in, 6
salivary gland enlargement, 76, 79, 84
Salmonella sp., 58, 83, 135–136, 143
salmonellosis, 48
salt, 13–14, 63. *See also* sodium
Sandoz Nutrition Corporation, 46
sanitation in food preparation and
    consumption, 124–133
scales, to measure body weight, 25–26
seafood, 16–17, 139, 140, 141
secretions as defense mechanisms, 6
"secretory" diarrhea, 58
seizures, 106
selenium, 9, 42, 178
  deficiencies in PWAs, 43
serum potassium, 170
sex, 157–158
  and energy expenditure, 22

depletion of
    during chronic diarrhea, 60
    during HIV infection, 31–32
  for esophagitis, 87
  from food sources compared with
    supplements, 32
  during pregnancy, 165–166
  recommended daily allowances for,
    31–32
  toxicity from megadoses, 34
  USDA dietary guidelines for, 12–13, 20
vomiting, 47, 76, 85
  as a drug side effect, 100, 102, 103, 104,
    106, 107
  as a symptom of foodborne illness, 135

W

warts, 78, 79, 81
washing
  cooking areas, 127–128, 131–133
  food, 130–131
  hands during food preparation, 126
wasting syndrome, 40, 42
water. *See also* dehydration
  deficiency from alcohol intake, 154
  extracellular, 40
  during foreign travel, 145
water activity, and microbial growth in food,
  119–121
water weight, 26, 40
weighing yourself, 24–28
weight, 12. *See also* weight loss
  maintaining, 22
  monitoring, 24–28
  relationship between energy intake and,
    22, 27
weight gain, during pregnancy, 165, 166
weight loss, 40, 81, 82
  causes of, 40–42, 106

and death, 38–40, 42–43
mechanism of, 42
nutritional management for, 107–108
prevention of, 47–49
and wasting compared with malnutrition,
  42–43
well-balanced diet, 11, 14
white blood cells, 99–100, 104
whole-body infections, 156
women, HIV infection in, 160–167
World Health Organization (WHO), 63–64
wound repair, 8

X

xerostomia, 41, 77, 79, 84, 85, 89
  as a drug side effect, 103, 109, 111
xylocaine, 85

Y

yeasts. *See also Candida* sp.
  classification of, 118, 134
  and food water activity scores, 120
  in gut flora, 58
yogurt, 17, 64, 71

Z

"zero-tolerance" hypothesis of alcohol
  intake, 149–150
zidovudine (AZT), 41, 97, 98, 99–101, 161,
  168–169
zinc, 8–9, 42, 90, 153
  body stores of, 60
  deficiencies in HIV-infected infants and
    children, 177
  deficiencies in PWAs, 43
  requirements during pregnancy, 165
Zovirax®, 80, 82, 100, 105